STRENGTHEN YOUR CORE

IMPROVE POSTURE

ENHANCE PERFORMANCE

STRENGTHEN FROM HEAD TO TOE

MARGARET MARTIN, PT, CSCS

KAMAJOJO PRESS

STRENGTHEN YOUR CORE

Improve Posture, Enhance Performance, Strengthen from Head to Toe
Margaret Martin, PT, CSCS

Photography: Richard Martin
Interior Design: Richard Martin
Video Production: Richard Martin

For information on getting permission for reprints and excerpts, contact Richard Martin at info@ melioguide.com.

Published in Canada by Kamajojo Press.
ISBN 978-0-9919125-0-6

Find us on the Web at www.melioguide.com/core

To report errors, please send a note to info@melioguide.com

Dedication

I dedicate this book to my Mom, Eliane Sylvain, who always believed in me, always supported my dreams, and always encouraged me to go out and play rather than help with housework. "It's clean underneath," she would say.

Remember this when prioritizing between putting your house or your body in shape!

Medical Advisory

Not all exercises or activities are suitable for everyone. If you have any medical issues that affect exercise such as diabetes, cardiac, or respiratory problems, then we strongly recommend that you consult with a licensed or certified health professional before engaging in an exercise program. If you feel any discomfort or pain during the exercise, stop.

Always seek the advice of your Physician, Physical Therapist, or other qualified health provider with any questions you may have regarding a medical condition or with reference to any content found in this book. Never disregard professional medical advice or delay in seeking it because of something you have read in this book.

The author is not responsible for any health problems that may result from training programs, products, or events you learn about through this book or her websites. If you engage in any exercise program you receive from this book or her websites, you agree that you do so at your own risk and are voluntarily participating in these activities.

Strengthen Your Core
Table of Contents

1. Introduction

Judy is 68 years old and has recently retired from her career as a librarian. She is very active, keenly interested in her health, and follows the latest research studies related to longevity, healthy aging, and fall reduction.

Unfortunately, arthritis and back pain limit Judy from doing all the things she wants to do. Whenever Judy takes the bus, the frequent stop-and-go movements aggravate her back and bring on her pain—causing her to wear a back brace.

Judy realizes that if she develops her own natural back brace, she would have less discomfort. She realizes she needs to strengthen her core.

Since Judy started working with me on a core strengthening exercise program that includes Plank and Side Plank poses, she has had a significant reduction in back pain from her frequent bus trips and she seldom wears her back brace.

Recently, Judy excitedly shared with me another benefit: "When I activate my core muscles my balance is much better!"

CORE BENEFITS

Like Judy, you too can strengthen your core. The benefits will be significant: reduced back pain, increased mobility, better posture, and an overall improvement in the quality of your life. But unfortunately, when many people think "strong core", they think washboard abs.

However, core strength goes beyond abdominals. Core strength incorporates the diaphragm, pelvic floor, and the muscles of the spine, the hips, and the shoulder. The Plank and Side Plank poses are the perfect prescription to build your core strength.

The Plank and Side Plank poses are beneficial for all types of individuals—from patients in rehabilitation to elite athletes in training. Both of these poses improve posture, and strengthen the muscles of the core and of the upper and lower body. When the correct pose is chosen and well executed, the benefits are numerous.

I am a Physical Therapist by training and profession. My clients range in age from 15 to 95. The 15 year old clients are usually sent my way for posture and performance-related issues. The many hours children (and adults) spend in a slouched forward position as they hover over their video games, smart phones, and computers can wreak havoc to the body. The 15 or 45 year old does not need more forward-bending movement in their lives. As a result, they certainly do not need crunches in their exercise program! This is why the Plank and Side Plank are so beneficial.

Many of my older clients have been diagnosed with osteoporosis or low bone density. In their quest to develop a stronger body, Planks and Side Planks allow us to build core strength while avoiding contraindicated crunches.

All of my clients benefit from doing Planks and Side Planks at a level that challenges them. Having taught so many variations of Planks and Side Planks over the years, I realized that knowledge and awareness of the different Plank and Side Plank progressions were not easily available—but needed to be. That is the motivation for me to write this book and develop *Building a Stronger Core*—the associated course for health and fitness professionals.

ABOUT THIS BOOK

This book is for someone concerned about their fitness and who wants to optimize their performance in a safe, efficient, and effective manner.

With this book, you will learn how to train your core safely. You will understand how you can modify the levers within your body to optimize and isolate the target of your training. In addition, you will understand the structures that are involved in core stabilization.

The early chapters provide you with information on anatomy, physiology, and the fundamentals of the Plank and Side Plank poses. After reading these chapters, you will better understand the modifications suggested for each of the poses.

I encourage you to visit my website where you will find instructional videos that accompany the content of this book. You will locate the video content at:

www.melioguide.com/core

After reading this book and reviewing the videos you will have:

» An understanding of the anatomical structures involved in doing Planks and Side Planks.

» An understanding of key elements needed to help you match your strengths and weaknesses with the most appropriate Plank and Side Plank poses for you.

» The knowledge you need to customize and progress your Plank and Side Plank as your fitness and functional strength improves.

» Multiple examples of Plank and Side Plank exercises from Beginner to Elite level.

TERMINOLOGY

The poses are identified as Plank 1, Plank 2, etc. This does not necessarily mean that Plank 2 will be easier than Plank 1. As you will learn, these poses involve all the musculature of your body, from your nose to your toes and so, depending on your strengths and weaknesses, the intensity of the exercise will change. That is the beauty of these exercises.

The Plank is a widely used term in Yoga, Pilates and fitness. The name *Side Plank* is not as widely known. In certain reference books, the *Side Plank* is also referred to as the *Side Bridge*—so the term is interchangeable.

Within the Side Plank, there are two angles that are covered when possible:

» The Side Plank—45 Degrees.

» The Side Plank—90 Degrees.

The Side Plank—45 Degrees has this name because you are turned 45 degrees away from the original Plank pose. With the Side Plank—90 Degrees, you are turned 90 degrees away from the original Plank pose. The Side Planks should be performed on both the right and left sides.

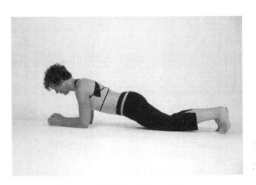

Figure 01.01. The Plank

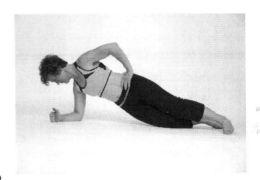

Figure 01.02.

The Side Plank—45 Degrees

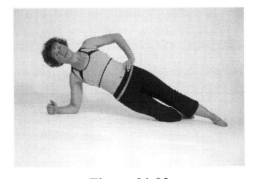

Figure 01.03.

The Side Plank—90 Degrees

2. Anatomy and Movement

*W*hen Peter was 32 years old, he experienced his first episode of back pain while playing a round of golf. Peter was halfway through a game when his back went into spasms. He had not done anything out of the ordinary to cause the back pains but they were so severe he was unable to finish his game. Since his first episode on the golf course, Peter had experienced regular flare-ups that usually lasted for as long as two weeks.

I first met Peter when he was 45 years old. I noticed during his assessment that he had a reversed breathing pattern, poor abdominal strength, and was very tight in his leg and trunk muscles. Peter also had poor body mechanics. After instructing him in diaphragmatic breathing, body mechanic training, and stretching, he gradually increased his flexibility and became more aware of all the triggers that caused his back pain to flare up.

However, once Peter became free of back pain, his commitment to continued therapy took lower priority compared to other things in his life. Those life priorities changed again when his garden and wood working projects came to a halt after his back pain reappeared!

Peter needed to strengthen his core.

This was a gradual process. Although Peter had been an avid cyclist, tennis, and basketball player through university and into his early 30s, he had gradually become more and more sedentary, fearful that he would worsen his pain.

Integrating core strength into an exercise routine gradually allowed him to bring his body back to its former shape. He has recently taken up tennis and cycling again, and has completed all his heavy woodworking and gardening projects without any set backs.

Part of Peter's rehab was to learn about the muscles of the core and how his posture impacted their function.

ANATOMY AND MOVEMENT

This chapter covers basic anatomy and physiology as they relate to the Plank and Side Plank poses. Specifically, the chapter contains a brief review of the anatomy of the spine, hip, and abdominal musculature. In addition, we will study the movements of the spine as they relate to finding a neutral spinal position. Video tutorials are located at www.melioguide.com/core to help the reader gain a better understanding of spinal movement.

The ability to hold a stable Plank and Side Plank is dependent on the coordination of all the muscles and ligaments surrounding the spine, hips, and shoulders, as well as the knees, ankles, elbows, and wrists. Therefore, the better you understand the information in this chapter, the easier it will be to make subtle adjustments to the poses. This will allow you to play with the components described in Chapter 3—Assess, Progress … Success!

Readers who do not have a background in anatomy may find parts of the chapter challenging. If necessary, you are encouraged to consult with your health or fitness professional.

ANATOMY OF STABILITY

Familiarity with the muscles involved in stability of the spine is core to creating a stronger Plank and Side Plank. When all the muscles work together, your inner core can be seen as a cylinder of pressure that sits in front of your spine. Your pelvic floor is at the bottom of the cylinder and your diaphragm is at the top. The walls of the core cylinder consist of the paraspinal muscles, the thoracolumbar and abdominal fascia, and the abdominal muscles.

Stability of the spine involves both active and passive stabilization. When you consciously activate certain muscles to stabilize your pose or posture, you are doing active stabilization. Passive stabilization, on the other hand, requires no conscious effort on your part. Passive stabilization involves bones and ligaments that are somewhat fixed in position and provide support without your conscious effort.

The key structures involved in active stabilization are reviewed to deepen your understanding and appreciation for their beauty and complexity.

ABDOMINALS

There are four abdominal muscles:

» Rectus abdominus.

» External oblique.

» Internal oblique.

» Transverse abdominus.

Each of these has connections to the abdominal fascia as illustrated in the diagram *Cross Section of the Abdominal Wall*. Together they work to create active stability around the spine.

THE ABDOMINAL FASCIA

The abdominal fascia connects the chest muscle (the pectoralis major) to the internal and external oblique muscles and surrounds the rectus abdominus as shown in the diagram *Anterior Torso Musculature and Abdominal Fascia*. The abdominal fascia allows forces to be transmitted around the abdomen.

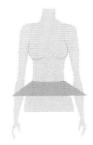

Abdominal Wall Cross Section

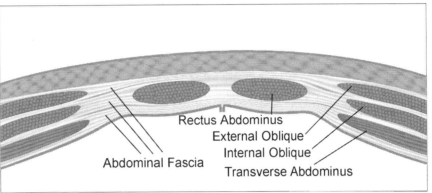

Rectus Abdominus
External Oblique
Internal Oblique
Abdominal Fascia
Transverse Abdominus

Figure 02.01. Cross Section of the Abdominal Wall

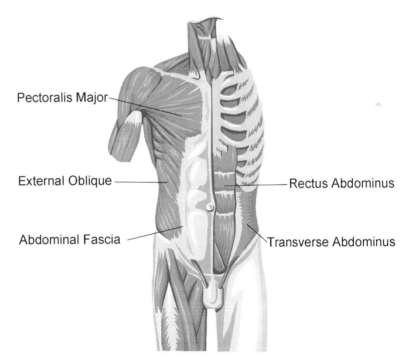

Pectoralis Major

External Oblique

Abdominal Fascia

Rectus Abdominus

Transverse Abdominus

Figure 02.02. Anterior Torso Musculature and Abdominal Fascia

THE THORACOLUMBAR FASCIA

The thoracolumbar fascia consists of three layers: the outer, middle, and inner layers. The outer layer of the thoracolumbar fascia (shown in the illustration *Posterior View of Torso*) is made up of tendinous fibers from the latissimus dorsi muscle. This allows the thoracolumbar fascia to act as a link between the arms and legs.

The middle and inner layers are attached to the transverse abdominus muscle. Acting as a unit, the fascia and abdominal muscles create what has been referred to as *nature's back belt*. I also refer to it as the *built in corset* when speaking to my older female clients.

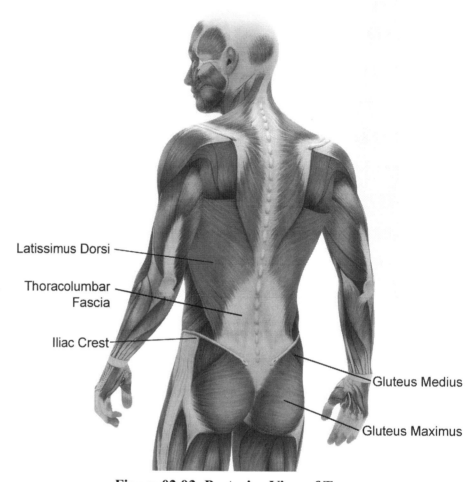

Figure 02.03. Posterior View of Torso

HIP MUSCULATURE

Muscles around the hips serve to transfer forces from the lower body to the pelvis and spine. The larger of the gluteal muscles include gluteus maximus and medius (also referred to as your buttocks). These are illustrated in the diagram *Posterior View of Torso*.

Weakness in these muscles becomes evident during single leg Planks and Side Planks since they are crucial in holding the pelvis level during single leg activities.

The psoas is a muscle commonly known as the hip flexor. It attaches to the lumbar spine and the femur. On its way to the femur it passes through the pelvis. It is an active stabilizer because it holds the lumbar spine to the pelvis.

THE PARASPINALS

The paraspinals are key muscles that enable an upright posture. For simplicity, we have divided the paraspinals into three groups.

The first paraspinals are the local muscle group composed of the rotatores and intertransversarii. These are short muscles that connect individual vertebrae together. They provide information to your brain regarding the position of each spinal unit and therefore play a critical role in your ability to feel the position of your spine.

The second group of paraspinal muscles are the multifidi. The multifidi are located in the lower back and cover two or three spinal levels. They are believed to work as local stabilizers.

The third group of paraspinals are the erector spinae group and consist of two long muscles located in the thoracic area (the mid-back). They have tendons that pass under the thoracolumbar fascia to attach to the pelvis and sacrum. They serve to protect and stabilize the lumbar spine but only when it is held in a neutral or extension position. When the lumbar spine is flexed, it is left without the protective action of the erector spinae and the spine is exposed to potentially damaging shear forces.

QUADRATUS LUMBORUM

This muscle, as the name implies, is quadrangular in shape and much wider than the muscles mentioned above. It is located in the lower back and connects the transverse process of the lumbar spine to the lower ribs and iliac crest of the pelvis. It works isometrically (without movement) and is an active stabilizer of the spine.

DIAPHRAGM

The diaphragm is the major muscle of respiration. It also makes up the roof of the inner core. It divides the space between your thoracic cavity and your abdominal cavity. It is sandwiched between your heart and lungs (above) and your stomach and liver (below).

The fibers of the diaphragm originate from the lower ribs and insert into the vertebral bodies of the lumbar spine (lower back). It has a key role as an active stabilizer—especially for power lifters.

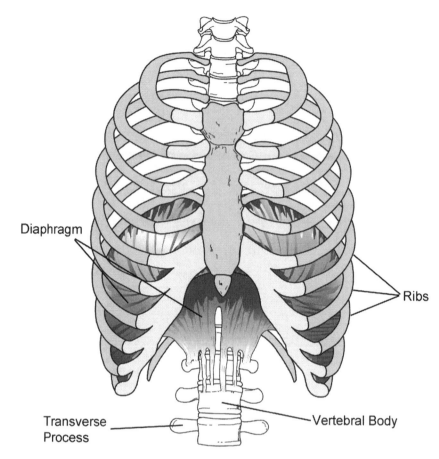

Figure 02.04. The Diaphragm

PELVIC FLOOR

The pelvic floor is the base of the inner core. It is especially important for men and women with weakened pelvic floors to involve the pelvic floor as part of the abdominal bracing. Failing to do so can lead to, or worsen, incontinence.

MOVEMENTS OF THE SPINE

The following undesirable movements of the lumbar spine (lower back) frequently occur with Planks and Side Planks and should be avoided:

» Flexion.

» Extension.

While performing Planks and Side Planks exercises, stability of the spine is key and it is critical that you establish and maintain good posture. Many individuals find it challenging to "sense" the position of their spine in a pose. This section describes how you can monitor and fine tune the position of your spine.

FLEXION

Flexion of the spine occurs when you slump forward. With your Planks and Side Planks, you are encouraged to flex from your hips and knees, and not your spine.

Here are the steps you can follow to develop awareness of your spine as you go into flexion:

» Start by sitting or standing tall.

» Slump forward and tilt your pelvis back as illustrated in the photo to the right.

» Notice how your lower back flattens (also known as flexion of the lumbar spine) and your shoulders and head fall forward.

» Go back to sitting or standing as tall as you can.

The photo to the right illustrates a Plank done with spinal flexion. The neutral position of the lumbar spine (lower back) is lost and the forward bend of the thoracic spine (mid-back) is exaggerated, resulting in your head falling forward out of alignment with your spine. For many, this is a habitual posture—one that should not be carried into your exercise routine.

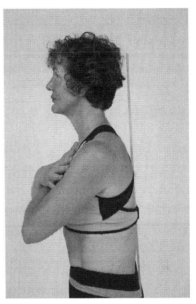

Figure 02.05.

Incorrect Form—Spinal Flexion

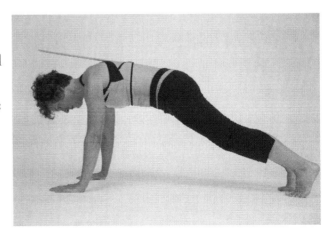

Figure 02.06.

Incorrect Form—Plank Done with Spinal Flexion

EXTENSION

Extension of the spine occurs when you reach up and arch back. An example of a back extension is the posture you take when you extend to paint a ceiling.

With your Planks and Side Planks, you are encouraged to maintain a neutral spine and avoid over extending your lumbar (lower) spine. The following steps will help you develop an awareness of the back bend or extension:

» Sit or stand with an elongated spine.

» Pull your shoulders as far back as you comfortably can and tilt your pelvis forward as illustrated in the photo to the right.

» Notice how your lower back arches (also known as extension of the lumbar spine).

» Go back to sitting or standing tall.

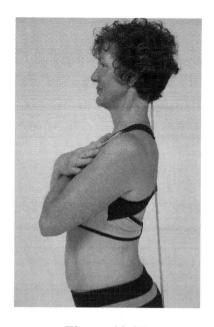

Figure 02.07.

Incorrect Form—Spinal Extension

The photo to the right illustrates a Plank done with spinal extension. The neutral position of the lumbar spine (lower back) is exaggerated and the forward bend of the thoracic spine (mid-back) is lost.

I often see this posture in individuals who "hang on their ligaments" for support rather than use their muscles. This is not encouraged.

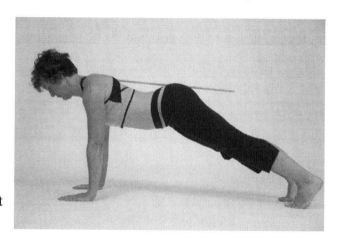

Figure 02.08.

Incorrect Form—Plank Done with Spinal Extension

ELONGATION OR AXIAL EXTENSION

Elongation, or axial extension of the spine, occurs when you elongate or lengthen the distance between your tailbone and the crown of your head. In drawing the crown of your head to the sky, you lengthen the natural curves of your spine and maintain a neutral lumbar spine. Doing so involves placing your lower back in a neutral position while lengthening the space between your lower ribs and pelvis. This is encouraged in developing a neutral spine position.

ESTABLISH A NEUTRAL SPINE POSITION

How to find your neutral spine position?

Pelvic rocking is a simple technique to determine the natural alignment of your lumbar spine. There are two starting positions I frequently use to help an individual explore their neutral lumbar spine position:

» Sit on a ball, or

» Lie supine with knees bent and feet resting on floor.

In either position, rock the pelvis forward and backward. The neutral position is located midway between the forward rocking limit (known as an anterior pelvic tilt) and the backward rocking limit (known as a posterior pelvic tilt). With some practice, you should feel both limits and then determine the neutral position.

The choice of which approach to use is dependent on which is more comfortable for you. The two options are presented below:

Option 1: Sit on a ball while maintaining your best postural alignment

» Make sure that you keep you posture aligned. You can achieve this by keeping the space between your breastbone and belly-button the same throughout the exercise. Do not slump forward.

» Push your tailbone out as though you are Donald Duck and then tuck in your tailbone as though you were the Pink Panther.

Option 2: Lie on your back

» Rock your pelvis back and forth.

» Flatten your lower spine (flexion) into the floor as much as you can then arch your lower spine (extension) off the floor as much as you can.

» Allow an exploration of the extremes of extension and flexion in the lumbar spine (lower back) by moving the arch of your back up and down.

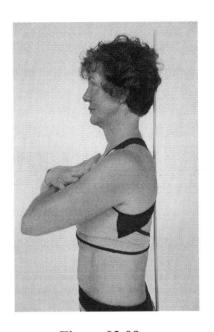

Figure 02.09.

Correct Form—Neutral Spine Position

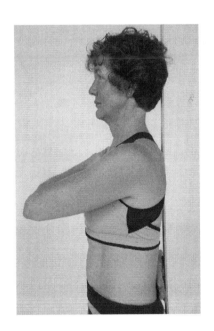

Figure 02.10.

Correct Form—A Neutral Spine Allows a Hand Space in Low Back

» Somewhere in between the two positions is your *neutral lumbar spine position*. You will have achieved it when you have an arch in your lower back that is approximately the width of your hand (as illustrated in the photos). This is the position you should strive to maintain with all the poses.

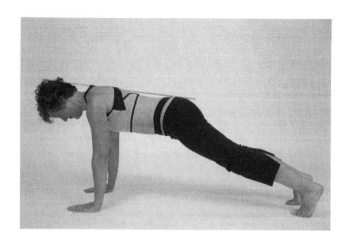

Figure 02.11.

Correct Form—Plank Done with Neutral Spine Position

BENDING FROM HIPS VERSUS THE SPINE

When getting into position for your Plank and Side Plank you should do so by bending, or hinging, from your hips rather than bending from your spine. Doing so will allow you to set your position before you increase the challenge on your shoulders, hips, and abdominals.

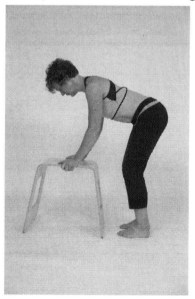

Figure 02.12.

Correct Form—Getting into the Plank by Bending at Your Hips

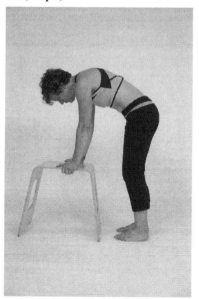

Figure 02.13.

Incorrect Form—Getting into the Plank by Bending at Your Spine

3. Assess, Progress ... Success!

*F*rom the age of 18 on, Robb experienced chronic back pain. He loved sports but recalls episodes of back and leg pain whenever he tried to play sports with his friends.

His worst episode occurred when he was 32 years old. While reaching into the car for his baby girl, he triggered the back spasms. The pain was so intense it caused him to fall to the ground.

By the time he was 34 years old, Robb knew that unless he committed time and energy to getting better, he would not be the active father he wanted to be.

An MRI showed an L4–5 disc bulge. Robb started following a therapeutic exercise program targeted at reducing his disc bulge and improving his strength and flexibility.

Once his back pain was under control, core strength became an integral part of Robb's conditioning program.

Along with Planks and Side Planks, Robb did overall body strengthening that included squats, lunges, and pushups. Even during periods when Robb got busy with life, he would always make time for his core work.

Now, in his early forties, Robb is able to keep up with his two active preteens and pursue new athletic activities.

Part of Robb's rehab was to allow him to continually improve his core strength to match his active lifestyle. For this he needed to understand all the variables he could modify to continually challenge himself. These variables are covered in the second half of this chapter, starting at "Progressing From A to E".

ASSESS, PROGRESS ... SUCCESS

Plank and Side Plank poses, when done properly, strengthen your core—but they also do so much more.

When looking for one or two exercises that allow you to target postural musculature, the neck extensors, side flexors, shoulder stabilizers, hip abductors, and ankle stabilizers, the Plank and Side Plank poses are the perfect prescription.

The Plank and Side Plank are frequently demonstrated on fitness and health websites and in a wide variety of print publications. They are a staple in many fitness classes. As a general rule, in fitness print and web publications and in exercise classes, only the more advanced level Plank and Side Plank poses are shown. I frequently find that fitness instructors and personal trainers overlook the natural progression from a Beginner or Active level to the advanced (Athletic and Elite) level Plank and Side Plank poses.

Frequently, individuals are encouraged to do advanced level Plank and Side Plank exercises without going through the necessary assessment and progression. As a result, many individuals attempt a Plank or Side Plank pose that is beyond their reach and invariably fail or learn to compromise their form.

Although most of the poses in this book are static, the progression is very dynamic.

ASSESS TO ENSURE SUCCESS

As mentioned previously, when properly matched with the capabilities of the individual, the Plank and Side Plank exercises are excellent for integrating stability and strength from our noses to our toes. Improperly matched, they can do more harm than good.

The key areas that need to be reviewed prior to starting the Plank and Side Plank exercises are:

1. Breathe from the diaphragm.

2. Activate the abdominal and pelvic floor musculature.

3. Optimize posture.

1. BREATHE FROM THE DIAPHRAGM

When you use your diaphragm correctly, you get more oxygen to your working muscles and you support the team of muscles that keeps your spine stable. This assists in your overall stability.

Breathing is an integral component of any exercise program. In order to achieve the full benefit from an exercise program, your breathing needs to be rhythmic and full.

How will I know if I am breathing with my diaphragm?

Follow these steps to determine whether you are using your diaphragm when you breathe:

» Breathe in through your nose and out through either your nose or mouth. Your breathing pattern should be natural and relaxed.

» Bring one hand to gently rest on the area of your abdomen just below your rib cage and above your belly button. You should feel your hand rise with each inhalation and fall with each exhalation.

» Now bring your hands to rest on either side of your lower rib cage. You should feel your ribs expand and your tummy rise as you inhale.

» When working on the core, many individuals find the coordination of the diaphragmatic breath and the contraction of the abdominals challenging. In order to reduce this challenge, focus on the breath into the lower ribs rather than into the abdominal area.

2. ACTIVATE ABDOMINAL AND PELVIC FLOOR MUSCULATURE

After taking a relaxed diaphragmatic breath, follow these tips as you exhale:

» Slowly and gently tighten your pelvic floor. The intensity should be mild. The analogy for women is to pretend to gently squeeze a tampon that is breakable. Men should feel a tightening of their perineal muscle, located in front of the anus and behind the genitals.

» Next, think about slowly and gently drawing your front pelvic bones together or your belly button towards your spine—without doing a pelvic tilt.

» Your goal is to tighten your abdominals with your back in a neutral position.

The Plank or Side Plank positions require the complete support of your abdominals. You should tighten the whole abdominal area while you execute the pose.

The following cues have been shown to be very helpful in eliciting the correct contraction:

» Women: Breath in … let it go … slowly, gently draw in your pelvic floor and lower tummy.

» Men: Breath in … let it go … slowly, gently draw up your scrotum and lower tummy.

Once the pelvic floor and the transverse abdominus are engaged, tighten your entire abdominal area.

3. OPTIMIZE POSTURE

The Plank and Side Plank are excellent for building postural muscle strength. However, to execute these exercises properly you need to make sure that you maintain proper (or optimal) postural alignment while performing each pose. Individuals who learn to hold a Plank or Side Plank in a undesirable position will take that position with them into all their day-to-day activities, strength training, and sports that require core strength.

If the Plank or Side Plank (or any exercise that you choose) makes your posture worse, then the intensity of the pose you have chosen is too great for your postural muscles. Respect this and go to an intensity that allows all your muscles to succeed!

How do you achieve optimal posture?

Good posture starts from the feet up. Follow these steps (pun intended) when doing any of the Plank poses:

» For Planks done from your feet, distribute your weight evenly through the ball of your foot with weight at the base of both your big toe and your little toe. This will ensure you keep your feet in neutral alignment. This foot placement is encouraged whether you practice your Plank with bare feet or shoes.

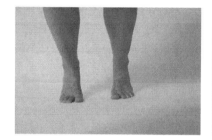 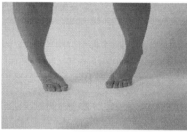 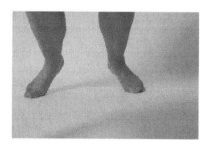

Figure 03.01.	**Figure 03.02.**	**Figure 03.03.**
Correct Foot Placement	**Incorrect Foot Placement**	**Incorrect Foot Placement**

» Keep your knee and hip joints soft (unlocked).

» Make sure your lumbar spine (lower back) is in a neutral position.

» Gently tighten your pelvic floor.

» Tighten your abdominals.

» Lengthen the space between your pelvis and your lower ribs.

» Gently tuck your shoulder blades downward and toward each other.

» Draw the crown of your head in the opposite direction from your tail bone.

PROGRESS, DON'T REGRESS

The three most common effects from improperly prescribed Planks and Side Planks are:

» **Discouragement and abandonment.** Attempts to do a pose that is too advanced can discourage anybody and cause them to prematurely abandon the pursuit of a strength training program. Assessment is ideal before embarking on a program that involves Plank or Side Plank poses. The most frequent problem I see with the Plank and Side Plank poses is that these exercises have been inappropriately prescribed or tried without an appropriate assessment. If you are using this book without the guidance of a health or fitness professional, I encourage you to start at the Beginner level and progress from Beginner Plank 1, 2, 3, etc until you reach a level that challenges you and allows you to keep optimum alignment as you perform the poses.

» **Undue discomfort, pain, and possibly strain.** I find that a number of people will persevere even though they find a Plank or Side Plank pose too challenging. A pose that is too intense can cause undue discomfort, pain and, possibly, a strain. In addition, I find that many people I see doing a Plank or Side Plank have been introduced to a variation of the exercise from a magazine. The model in the magazine or on a web site may be doing the pose with correct form, but too often, the pose is too intense for the reader.

» **Engagement of the wrong muscles.** An individual who attempts a Plank or Side Plank pose before they are ready will engage muscles that were not intended to be used in that exercise. This forces other muscles (that were not the original targets of the exercise) to provide support. The result: a compensatory, less stable position is learned and reinforced.

This book presents over seventy Plank and Side Plank poses. Suggestions for gentler and more challenging variations are included. A good understanding of the components covered in the next section will allow you to create over one hundred different poses.

PROGRESSING FROM A TO E

It is better to master a level that is just below your full challenge level and build from there. The following variables, referred to as the A, B, C, D, and E's of the Plank and Side Plank, provide you with the tools you need to make adjustments to any pose.

A: ANTHROPOMETRIC MEASUREMENTS

The height and weight of an individual can have a significant impact on the intensity of the exercise. Someone who is six feet tall (or taller) will have a more significant load on their core when they hold a pose compared to someone who is five feet tall. The longer lever arm (in the taller individual) incrementally increases the load. Individuals who are heavier will require more strength to maintain a pose. Finally, how the individual's weight is distributed can affect how challenging they find the pose.

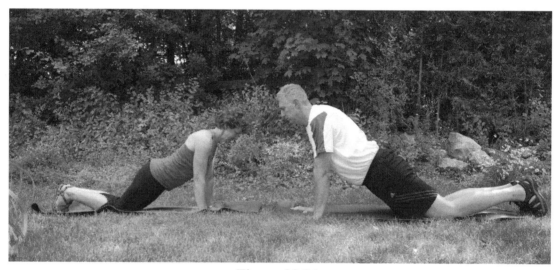

Figure 03.04.

Longer Lever Arm Increases the Load
Me on Left (5' 2") and Peter on Right (6' 7")

B: BODY ANGLE

Several angles need to be considered when contemplating the perfect Plank or Side Plank. These include:

» The angle created from the knees (or feet, depending on the pose), up through the hips, shoulder, and head. The more horizontal the body (the smaller the angle), the greater the resistance required by all the musculature to hold against gravity. The more vertical the body is (the greater the angle), the less effect gravity will have. A greater body angle will reduce the load on the shoulders and neck.

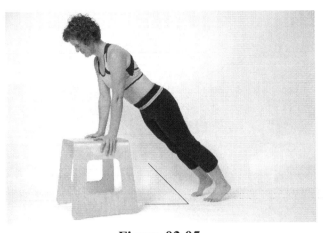

Figure 03.05.

Greater Body Angle =
Reduced Shoulder and Abdominal Loading

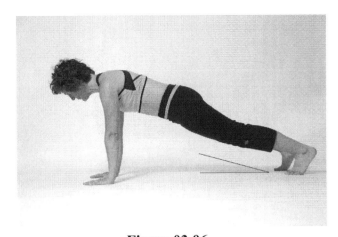

Figure 03.06.

Lesser Body Angle =
Increased Shoulder and Abdominal Loading

» The angle created at the shoulders is another variable that should be considered. The greater the angle, the greater the demand on the shoulder joint. An increased shoulder angle will also increase the demand on the shoulder and the core musculature. It can be an effective way to intensify a pose but should be only done when an individual has the shoulder strength to do so safely.

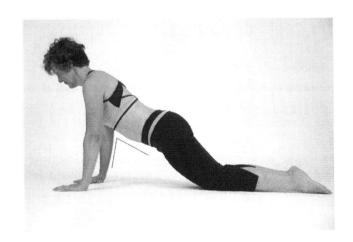

Figure 03.07.

Lesser Shoulder Angle =
Reduced Shoulder and Abdominal Loading

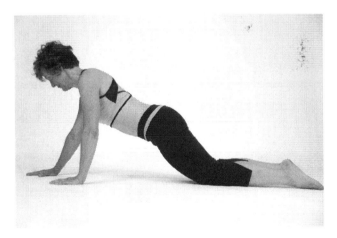

Figure 03.08.

Greater Shoulder Angle =
Increased Shoulder and Abdominal Loading

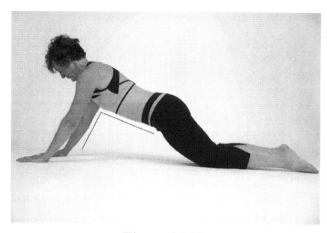

Figure 03.09.

**Greater Shoulder Angle =
Increased Shoulder and Abdominal Loading**

» Most Plank and Side Plank positions are performed with your shoulder, hip, knee, and ankle aligned (as illustrated in the left photo below). However, raising the hips allows the individual to adjust the intensity of the plank.

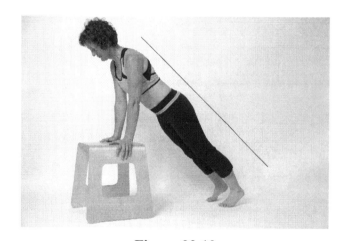

Figure 03.10.

Straight Hips = Increased Abdominal Loading

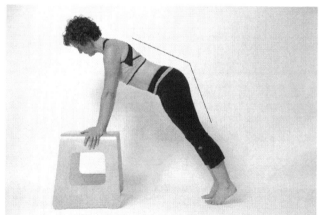

Figure 03.11.

Higher Hips = Reduced Abdominal Loading

» The angle created at the hip joint during a Side Plank is another variable that allows the intensity of the Side Plank to be modified in real time. Muscular analysis of the Side Plank shows more activity in all the abdominal muscles when the thighs and knees are in line with the torso in comparison to doing the same level Side Plank with your knees and thighs in front of your torso.

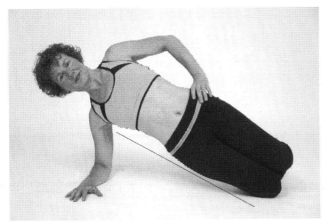

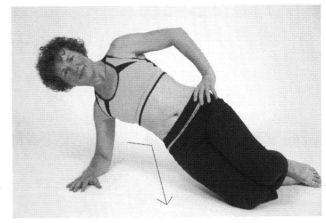

Figure 03.12.

Figure 03.13.

Straight Knees = Increased Abdominal Loading   **Knees Forward = Reduced Abdominal Loading**

C: CONTACT AREA AND STABILITY

The stability of the *surface* and amount of *surface area* at the point of contact allows endless modifications to a Plank and Side Plank. It is advisable to start on a stable surface such as a wall, a chair, a step, or the floor. In order to increase the challenge to your core and shoulder musculature, you can move the pose to an unstable surface.

The more unstable the surface under your points of contact, the more challenging the pose will be. Examples of progression include foam, foam roller, wobble board, Bosu, exercise ball, medicine ball, and suspension trainers. Moving the Plank and Side Plank onto unstable surfaces (as shown below) is great for the deeper joint stabilizers of the hip, knees, ankles, shoulders, and spine. Movement of an arm or leg can add variety and challenge to any of the Planks or Side Planks.

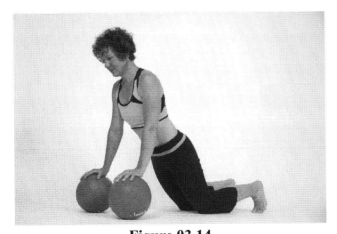

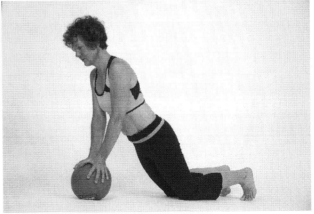

Figure 03.14.

Figure 03.15.

Two Medicine Balls

One Medicine Ball

The smaller the point of contact surface area, the more intense the pose will be. Further, when imposed upon an unstable surface such as the exercise or medicine ball, you can make adjustments to the intensity of poses in real time by rolling the balls.

A pose on one foot will be more challenging than the same pose performed on two feet. A pose with feet together will be more challenging than a pose with feet hip-width apart.

During a recent workshop, one of the participants was surprised that she could hold a Plank with both her hands and feet on the floor but she was unable to maintain her pose when she had her hands on a chair and she attempted to raise one leg. With her hands on a chair, the Plank should have been significantly easier for her. However, she had weakness around her hip joints which made lifting one foot and the hold more challenging for her.

Individuals who find weight-bearing through their wrist intolerable should be progressed through the forearm support positions.

Clothing can also make a difference. For beginners, clothing that is smooth and slippery on points of contact can increase the level of difficulty. Spandex pants can cause instability at the hips and knees (assuming that the knees are a point of contact). Socks can also cause instability at the feet.

Finally, the ***choice of footwear*** can affect stability. Rubber soled shoes will provide a greater level of stability for poses performed from the feet. Therefore, performing a pose in bare feet can increase the challenge by reducing the stability at the point of contact. Individuals with arthritic toes will find the use of rubber soled shoes very beneficial.

D: DISTANCE

The greater the distance between the point of contact and the core, the greater the challenge experienced during the exercise. For example, a Plank from the feet will be more demanding than a Plank done from the knees. Planks and Side Planks utilize the body's lever system to vary the resistance.

In his book, *Essence of Stability Ball Training*, Juan Carlos Santana progresses a pushup using the following distance-related intensity progressions. In each case, hands are on the floor:

» Exercise ball under the hips.

» Exercise ball under the thighs.

» Exercise ball under the knees.

» Exercise ball under the shins.

» Exercise ball under the feet.

These progressions are equally applicable to the Plank. After all a pushup, when well executed, is a Plank in motion.

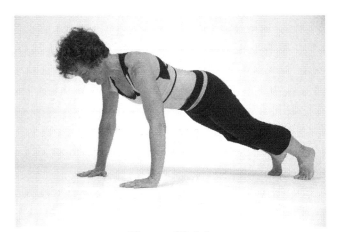

Figure 03.16.

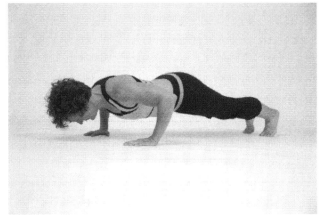

Figure 03.17.

A Pushup is a Plank in Motion

E: EFFORT

Your choice of Plank and Side Plank is dependent on your therapeutic goals. Are you choosing the Plank or Side Plank to increase ankle stability, add variety to a shoulder stabilization program, or simply to challenge the core?

Performing a Plank from your hands (straight arms) will challenge upper body musculature more than doing it through the forearms. Straight arms will engage the forearm muscles and triceps and place a greater load on the shoulder stabilizers.

Although the Plank and Side Plank poses are often prescribed as exercises for transverse and oblique abdominals, they are also effective exercises to address other joints that may need attention. For example, an individual who has mastered a Plank on two feet but who has weakness in their hips or ankles could be challenged to progress to a single leg Plank as part of their conditioning program.

Lastly, the Plank or Side Plank should *NOT* elicit strain in the back. The strain should be on the abdominal muscles. If there is any back strain while doing the pose, the hold time can be reduced, the hips can be raised, or a more appropriate pose should be selected.

If back discomfort persists, stop. Reevaluate the technique to ensure that the correct muscles are being used. Many people manage to do the Plank by activating muscles other than those originally intended which means the benefit is lost and the back becomes strained.

4. Frequently Asked Questions

Individuals have many questions when they are introduced to the Plank and Side Plank poses. Instead of distributing them around the various chapters, I decided the questions needed a chapter dedicated to them. Here they are.

1. WHERE DO I START?

This book is written in such a manner that, by starting at the beginning of the book, you will have the tools you need to begin a Plank or Side Plank safely by the time you reach the exercise section. At the beginning of each exercise chapter, guidance is provided to assist you in determining whether that level is suitable for you.

2. WHAT TYPE OF WARMUP SHOULD I DO?

If your Planks or Side Planks are done at the end of your exercise routine, you have already warmed up. If the poses are being done by themselves, then I would encourage you to do Beginner level Planks in order to prepare the body for the more advanced level Planks. If you are a Beginner level, spend a few minutes on your hands and knees to prepare your body. Crawling is also an excellent warmup activity.

3. HOW MANY REPETITIONS OF EACH EXERCISE SHOULD I DO?

The Plank and Side Planks are most often performed as static holds. With the Plank or Side Plank, you are working on endurance. Build your endurance in the following way:

» 5 second hold; repeat six times.

» 10 second hold; repeat three times.

- » 15 second hold; repeat two times.
- » 30 second hold once.
- » 30 second hold; repeat two times.
- » 30 second hold; repeat three times.

Endurance athletes will benefit from increasing hold-times up to three minutes.

4. HOW DO I KNOW WHEN TO PROGRESS?

When you are able to easily perform three consecutive 30 second holds (with 30 second rest-times between each hold), you can consider the next challenge level. You can also gradually reduce your rest time to intensify the challenge.

Success at each step is how you ensure safe progression. If in doubt, always err on the side of caution. Better to master a level that is just below your full challenge level than to struggle with a pose.

5. HOW FREQUENTLY SHOULD PLANKS AND SIDE PLANKS BE DONE?

Planks and Side Planks need not be part of an exercise program more than twice weekly. They should be kept to the end of an exercise routine so that the abdominals are not fatigued before executing other exercises that might be in need of their support.

However, if certain Plank and Side Plank poses have become easy for you, then you can incorporate them into a daily routine.

6. WHAT SHOULD BE MY POSITIONING?

- » Place your hands/elbows directly under your shoulder joint.
- » Draw your shoulders blades gently downward and toward each other.
- » Maintain a natural inward curve in the small of your back and in your neck. This is referred to as a neutral spine.
- » If your arms are extended, keep your elbows joints "soft" or unlocked.
- » If your legs are extended, keep your knee joints "soft" or unlocked.

7. CAN I DO EXERCISES FROM DIFFERENT LEVELS?

Ab-solutely! Depending on your strengths and weaknesses you may do Planks and Side Planks from different levels during the same workout. This is common in individuals who have weakness around either the shoulder or hip.

The Plank poses involve weight-bearing across hands or forearms, and knees or feet. If you have weakness in one side, the other can compensate for it.

The Side Planks involve weight-bearing through one hand or forearm, and one knee or foot. If you have weakness at the hip, shoulder, wrist, or foot, the corresponding Side Plank will become much more difficult and you may have to do a lower level Side Plank to build up.

8. HOW CAN I REDUCE STRAIN ON MY WRISTS?

Many people are not used to putting a lot of weight through their wrists. The following are some tips to reduce the strain on your wrists.

» When your hands are on the ball, keep your fingers pointing toward the floor.

» Spread your fingers wide and ensure that you have weight through the knuckle of the index and little finger. When appropriate, also grip with the tips of all your fingers. This helps distribute the weight off your wrists and into your entire hand.

» When your hands are on the wall, a step, chair, or floor, place a folded facecloth under the fleshy part of your hands so as to reduce the amount of bend at the wrist. Use dumbbells or push up bars as a hand support to reduce wrist bending.

» When working from the wall, step chair, or floor, you can bear weight through your knuckles and keep the wrists in a neutral position.

» If weight-bearing through the wrists or hands is too uncomfortable, regardless of the above tips, I suggest you do the Planks and Side Planks from your forearms.

9. HOW CAN I REDUCE STRAIN ON MY SHOULDERS?

As you enter into every Plank and Side Plank you should set your shoulders by gently drawing your shoulder blades downward and toward each other.

In addition, while performing the Side Plank, the free hand can either rest on the surface or over the supporting shoulder.

10. SHOULD I FEEL PAIN IN THE BACK?

Many people look for therapeutic, exercise-based ways to reduce their back pain. In their quest to get stronger and fitter (and reduce the repeated occurrence of back pain), they turn to exercises such as the Plank or Side Plank.

These exercises are a great choice but it is imperative that *NO* strain is felt in the back. The strain should be felt in the abdominal muscles.

11. WILL I BENEFIT FROM TRAINING MY CORE IF I HAVE BACK PAIN?

Just to set the record straight: not everyone will have a reduction in back pain by working on his or her core musculature, but they will have improved function. At the same time, you should not have any increase in your back pain when doing a Plank or Side Plank.

12. IF I AM RECOVERING FROM BACK PAIN, SHOULD I HOLD AS LONG AS INDICATED IN QUESTION 3?

In Dr. McGill's book, *Low Back Disorders*, recommended hold-time for poses such as the Plank and Side Plank is limited to 7–8 seconds in cases of rehabilitation of low back disorders. This recommendation is a result of a study showing that oxygen deprivation to the muscles occurs after holding an isometric contraction (squeezing a muscle without movement) for more than 8 seconds. More frequent repetitions rather than one longer hold might be considered if you are recovering from a low back disorder.

13. WHAT ARE THE CHALLENGES TO DEVELOPING CORE STRENGTH?

There are many challenges to developing core strength. Some of them include:

» **History of back pain.** Individuals who have had recurrent back pain will find that their abdominals have a harder time to work. This inhibition can be overcome with appropriate progression.

» **History of abdominal/back surgery.** An assault to the abdominal or back musculature can lead to inhibition of the musculature.

» **Core exercises that are too intense and force you to compromise your form.** In an attempt to keep up with a class or to try a pose from a magazine, an individual whose core musculature is not prepared for the level of difficulty will be forced to compensate and recruit alternative muscles. This learned pattern can become ingrained. Further, poor form usually requires more time to unlearn than to teach proper form in the first place.

» **Diastasis Recti.** The condition that occurs when the connective tissue between the rectus abdominus muscles becomes overstretched and weakened is known as *Diastasis Recti*. The more the connective tissue stretches sideways, the thinner and weaker it becomes. It can occur in the second or third trimester of pregnancy or when someone is obese. Individuals with diastasis recti may benefit from wearing a specific waist belt to encourage the connective tissue to regain its connectivity. If you have been diagnosed with diastasis recti, you are encouraged to seek guidance from a health professional.

14. WHAT DO YOU THINK OF CRUNCHES (SITUPS)?

For individuals in Martial Arts or other sports that require a strong rectus abdominus, the simple curlup can be performed rather than the crunch (or situp). In the curlups, the head and shoulders lift off the floor but the lower part of the shoulder blades remain in contact with the floor.

Individuals with osteoporosis or a history of disc herniation should not be doing crunches or curlups.

In our modern culture we spend far too much time slouched over our laptops and iPhones. The precious little time we spend on exercise should focus on creating a balance to what we do all day long. I encourage you to shift the time spent doing crunches to doing Planks and Side Planks.

15. HOW DOES CORE TRAINING ENHANCE PERFORMANCE?

If an individual is unable to hold a pose with good form, I can guarantee that he or she will be using the same poor or compensatory form in their other activities, sports, and exercises.

Likewise, if an individual maintains a strong, well-aligned posture during their pose, they will likely take that alignment into their sports and enhance their performance.

16. DO YOU RECOMMEND OTHER EXERCISES TO STRENGTHEN THE CORE?

Yes, the Plank and Side Plank should not be seen as the only exercises to strengthen the core. Much research advocates not only isometric but also dynamic training to stimulate and develop all the muscles involved in core training. However, the Plank and Side Plank can be seen as building blocks to dynamic strength.

17. DO YOU HAVE TRAINING FOR HEALTH AND FITNESS PROFESSIONALS?

Yes. We have an online course for fitness and health care professionals called *Building a Stronger Core*. If you are interested in further training in this area, please visit www.melioguide.com/plank.

5. Beginner Plank Poses

Planks are always easier than Side Planks and should be explored first. In a Plank, you distribute your weight through both shoulders, as well as the arms and wrists. For individuals getting back into shape, this is the safest route to start. The Beginner level Planks are appropriate for individuals who are de-conditioned or recovering from injury.

I encourage you to ensure that all foundational elements in Chapter 3 are considered prior to exploring the poses. That chapter covers your breath, posture, and abdominal musculature—all essential elements to supporting your pose.

Hold times, repetitions, and training frequency are covered in Chapter 4—Frequently Asked Questions.

As you enter into every Plank, you should set your shoulders by gently drawing your shoulder blades downward and toward each other.

BEGINNER PLANK 1

FOREARMS AGAINST WALL, FEET ON FLOOR

» Stand tall and place your forearms shoulder-width apart, just below shoulder-height, against a wall.

» Lean into your forearms.

» Step back and bring your feet hip-width apart and parallel to one another.

» Lower your hips.

» Endeavour to keep your body in a straight line and your head in line with your body.

» Hold.

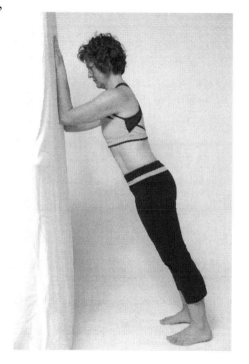

Challenging Variation:

» Follow the above steps but use your hands instead of your forearms for support.

BEGINNER PLANK 2

FOREARMS ON COUNTER TOP, FEET ON FLOOR

» Stand tall and place your forearms shoulder-width apart, just below shoulder-height, against a counter top or tall table.

» Lean into your forearms.

» Step back and bring your feet hip-width apart and parallel to one another.

» Lower your hips.

» Endeavour to keep your body in a straight line and your head in line with your body.

» Hold.

Safety Recommendation:

» If you have had low back pain in the past, keep your hips raised slightly towards the ceiling. Once you have mastered this level without any strain on your back, drop your hips and bring them in line with your body.

Challenging Variation #1:

» Follow the above steps but use your hands instead of your forearms for support.

Challenging Variation #2:

» Follow the directions listed above except use a lower surface for support (the third step in stairwell or the back of a sofa works well).

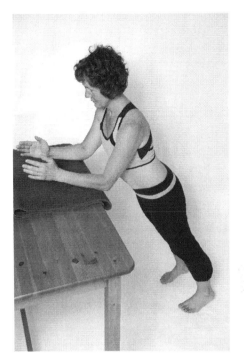

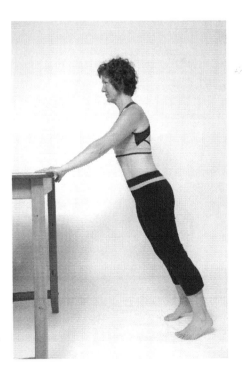

BEGINNER PLANK 3

HANDS ON BALL WITH BALL RESTING ON SOFA, FEET ON FLOOR

» Place a burst resistant exercise ball on your sofa or chair. The ball should be just an inch or so from the back of the chair—to allow you to rest into it, if necessary.

» Place your hands shoulder-width apart and at an equal distance from the center of the ball.

» Lean into your hands.

» Step back and bring your feet hip-width apart and parallel to one another.

» Lower your hips.

» Endeavour to keep your body in a straight line and your head in line with your body.

» Hold.

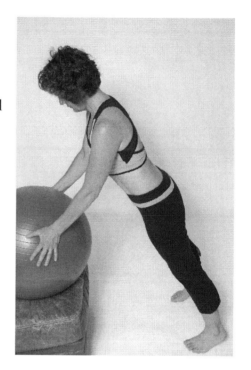

Gentler Variation #1:

» Allow the ball to rest into the back of the chair/sofa. This way you only have to work on side-to-side instability rather than multidirectional instability.

Gentler Variation #2:

» Place the ball against the wall with your fingers pointing towards the wall and just below shoulder-height.

Challenging Variation:

» In a controlled manner, move the ball 2 inches to the right and then 2 inches to the left.

BEGINNER PLANK 4

HANDS ON FLOOR, PELVIS RESTING ON BALL

» Kneel tall behind a burst resistant ball The ideal ball size is one in which your thighs are parallel to the floor when you are sitting on it.

» Lower yourself onto the ball and then firmly press your hands into the floor.

» Walk out on your hands until the ball is rests under your pelvis.

» Endeavour to keep your body in a straight line and your head in line with your body.

» Hold.

» Carefully walk your hands back to your start position.

A
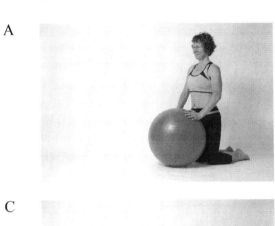

B
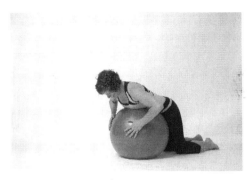

C
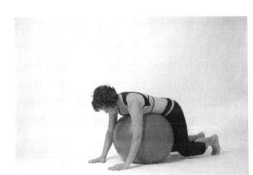

D
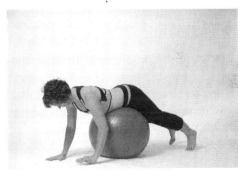

E
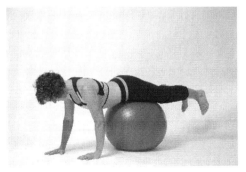

Safety Recommendation:

» Create a valley with your bed or sofa on one side of you and cushions on the other side. This will provide bumpers for you to maintain control of the ball.

BEGINNER PLANK 5

HANDS ON FLOOR, UPPER THIGHS RESTING ON BALL

» Kneel tall behind a burst resistant ball. The ideal ball size is one in which your thighs are parallel to the floor when you are sitting on it.

» Lower yourself onto the ball and press your hands firmly and evenly into the floor.

» Walk out on your hands until the ball rests under your upper thighs.

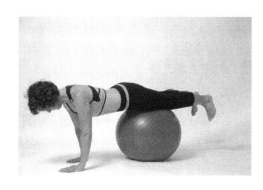

» Tighten your abdominals as soon as your pelvis leaves the ball so as not to have your low back sag towards the floor.

» Endeavour to keep your body in a straight line and your head in line with your body.

» Hold.

» Carefully walk your hands back to your start position.

Safety Recommendation:

» Create a valley with your bed or sofa on one side of you and cushions on the other side. This will provide bumpers for you to maintain control of the ball.

Challenging Variation:

» Place your hands in a staggered position during your hold.

» Alternate lead hands.

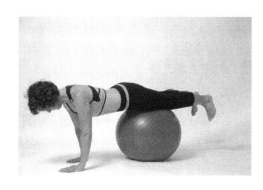

BEGINNER PLANK 6

HANDS ON FLOOR, UPPER THIGHS RESTING ON BALL WITH WEIGHT SHIFT

» Kneel tall behind a burst resistant ball. The ideal ball size is one in which your thighs are parallel to the floor when you are sitting on it.

» Lower yourself onto the ball and press your hands firmly and evenly into the floor.

» Walk out on your hands until the ball rests under your upper thighs.

» Tighten your abdominals as soon as your pelvis leaves the ball so as not to have your low back sag towards the floor.

» Endeavour to keep your body in a straight line and your head in line with your body.

» Transfer 80% of your weight onto one thigh. (Lifting one leg off is a later progression.)

» Hold for 2 to 3 seconds, alternating sides.

» Carefully walk back to your start position.

Safety Recommendation:

» Create a valley with your bed or sofa on one side of you and cushions on the other side. This will provide bumpers for you to maintain control of the ball.

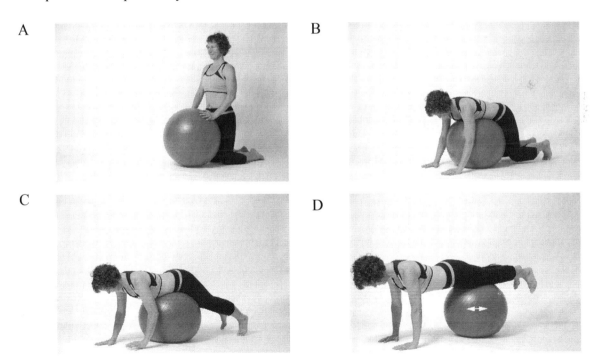

A   B   C   D

BEGINNER PLANK 7

FOREARMS ON CHAIR, KNEES ON FLOOR

» Kneel tall and place your forearms shoulder-width apart against a chair.

» Move your knees back.

» Lower your hips.

» Endeavour to keep your body in a straight line and your head in line with your body.

» Hold.

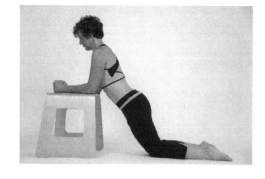

Safety Recommendation:

» If you have had low back pain in the past, keep your hips raised slightly toward the ceiling. Once you have mastered this level without any strain on your back, drop your hips and bring them in line with your body.

6. Beginner Side Plank Poses

Side Planks are always more challenging than Planks. They require more strength through the shoulder, elbow, and wrist on the supporting side. They also require more strength through the lateral musculature of the torso, hips, and ankles.

The Beginner level Planks are appropriate for individuals who are de-conditioned or recovering from injury.

I encourage you to explore the Plank poses first to allow you to estimate the intensity of your Side Plank.

The Side Planks are labelled either Side Plank (number)—45 Degrees or Side Plank (number)—90 Degrees. A Side Plank (number)—45 Degrees identifies the position as midway between a Plank and a Side Plank (number)—90 Degrees.

As you enter into every Side Plank, you should set your shoulders by gently drawing your shoulder blades downward and toward each other.

In addition, while performing the Side Plank, the free hand can either rest on the surface or over the supporting shoulder.

BEGINNER SIDE PLANK 1—45 DEGREES

FOREARM AGAINST WALL, FEET ON FLOOR

» Stand tall with your shoulders at a 45 degree angle from the wall.

» Place one forearm on the wall just below shoulder height.

» Lean into your forearm.

» Step away from the wall as indicated in the photo.

» Lower your hips.

» Endeavour to keep your body in a straight line and your head in line with your body.

» Hold.

» Switch sides.

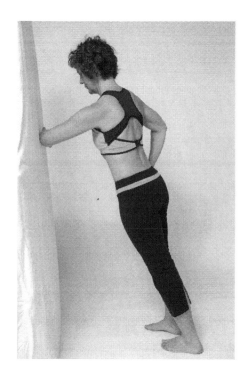

Safety Recommendation:

» If you are not accustomed to putting weight through one arm, consider keeping the other hand on the wall for additional support until you build more shoulder strength.

Challenging Variation:

» Follow the steps listed above except use your hand for support and not your forearm.

BEGINNER SIDE PLANK 1—90 DEGREES

FOREARM AGAINST WALL, FEET ON FLOOR

» Stand tall sideways from the wall.

» Place one forearm on the wall just below shoulder height.

» Lean into your forearm.

» Step away from the wall as indicated in the photo.

» Place your feet parallel to the wall. When your left arm is supporting you, your right foot will be the leading foot and vice versa.

» Lower your hips.

» Endeavour to keep your body in a straight line and your head in line with your body.

» Hold.

» Switch sides.

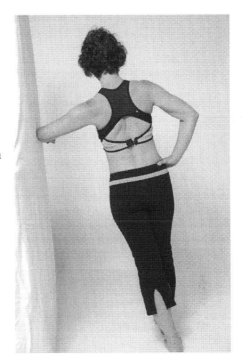

Challenging Variation:

» Follow the steps listed above except use your hand for support and not your forearm.

BEGINNER SIDE PLANK 2—45 DEGREES

FOREARMS ON COUNTERTOP, FEET ON FLOOR

» Stand tall at a 45 degree angle from the countertop.

» Place one forearm on the countertop.

» Lean into your forearm.

» Step away from the counter as indicated in the photo.

» Lower your hips.

» Endeavour to keep your body in a straight line and your head in line with your body.

» Hold.

» Switch sides.

Safety Recommendation:

» If you are not accustomed to putting weight through one arm, consider keeping the other hand on the countertop for additional support until you build more shoulder strength.

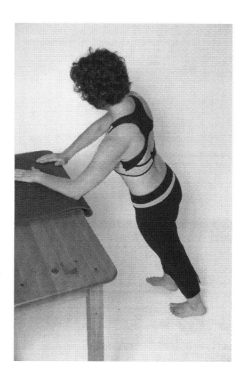

BEGINNER SIDE PLANK 2—90 DEGREES

FOREARMS ON COUNTERTOP, FEET ON FLOOR

» Stand tall sideways from the countertop.

» Place one forearm on the countertop.

» Lean into your forearm.

» Step away from the countertop as indicated in the photo.

» Place your feet parallel to the countertop. When your left arm is supporting you, your right foot will be the leading foot and vice versa.

» Lower your hips.

» Endeavour to keep your body in a straight line and your head in line with your body.

» Hold.

» Switch sides.

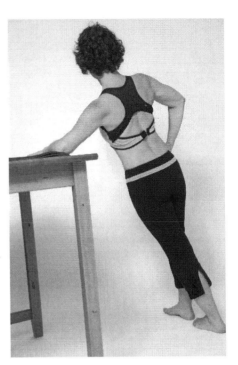

BEGINNER SIDE PLANK 3—45 DEGREES

HAND ON COUNTERTOP, FEET ON FLOOR

» Stand tall at a 45 degree angle from the countertop.

» Place one hand on the countertop.

» Lean into your hand.

» Step away from the counter as indicated in the photo.

» Lower your hips.

» Endeavour to keep your body in a straight line and your head in line with your body.

» Hold.

» Switch sides.

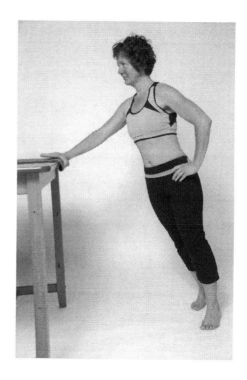

Safety Recommendation:

» If you are not accustomed to putting weight through one arm, consider keeping the other hand on the countertop for additional support until you build more shoulder strength.

BEGINNER SIDE PLANK 3—90 DEGREES

HAND ON COUNTERTOP, FEET ON FLOOR

» Stand tall sideways from the countertop.

» Place one hand on the countertop.

» Lean into your hand.

» Step away from the counter as indicated in the photo.

» Place your feet parallel to the wall. When your right arm is supporting you, your left foot will be the leading foot and vice versa.

» Lower your hips.

» Endeavour to keep your body in a straight line and your head in line with your body.

» Hold.

» Switch sides.

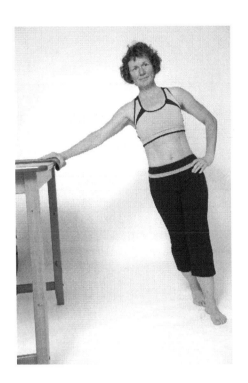

BEGINNER SIDE PLANK 4—45 DEGREES

FOREARM ON CHAIR, RESTING ON SIDE OF KNEE (LOWER LEG), BOTTOM KNEE BENT, TOP KNEE STRAIGHT

» Kneel tall at a 45 degree angle away from the chair.

» Place one forearm on the chair with your shoulder directly over your elbow.

» Lean into your forearm as you straighten your top (opposite) leg.

» Push through your top foot to move your bottom knee away from the chair.

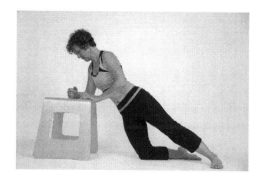

» Lower your hips.

» Endeavour to keep your body in a straight line and your head in line with your body.

» Hold.

» Switch sides.

Safety Recommendation:

» If you are not accustomed to putting weight through one arm, consider keeping the other hand on the chair for additional support until you build more shoulder strength.

BEGINNER SIDE PLANK 4—90 DEGREES

FOREARM ON CHAIR, RESTING ON SIDE OF KNEE (LOWER LEG), BOTTOM KNEE BENT, TOP KNEE STRAIGHT

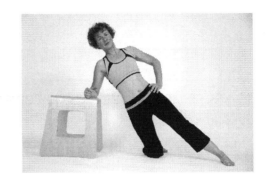

» Kneel tall sideways from the chair.

» Place one forearm on the chair with your shoulder directly over your elbow.

» Lean into your forearm as you straighten your top (opposite) leg.

» Push through your top foot to move your bottom knee away from the chair.

» Lower your hips.

» Endeavour to keep your body in a straight line and your head in line with your body.

» Hold.

» Switch sides.

BEGINNER SIDE PLANK 5—45 DEGREES

FOREARM ON 2ND STEP, RESTING ON SIDE OF KNEE (LOWER LEG), BOTTOM KNEE BENT, TOP KNEE STRAIGHT

» Kneel at a 45 degree angle away from a step.

» Place one forearm on the step with your shoulder directly over your elbow.

» Lean into your forearm as you straighten your top (opposite) leg.

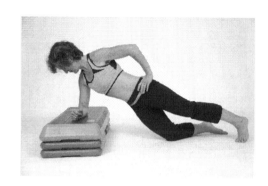

» Push through your top foot to move your bottom knee away from the step.

» Lower your hips.

» Endeavour to keep your body in a straight line and your head in line with your body.

» Hold.

» Switch sides.

Safety Recommendation:

» If you are not accustomed to putting weight through one arm, consider keeping the other hand on the step for additional support until you build more shoulder strength.

Challenging Variation:

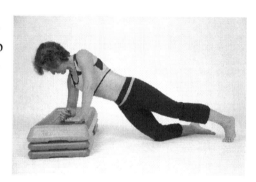

» Follow the directions listed above except use the first step in stairwell for support.

BEGINNER SIDE PLANK 5—90 DEGREES

FOREARM ON 1ST OR 2ND STEP, RESTING ON SIDE OF KNEE (LOWER LEG), BOTTOM KNEE BENT, TOP KNEE STRAIGHT

» Kneel sideways from a step.

» Place one forearm on the step with your shoulder directly over your elbow.

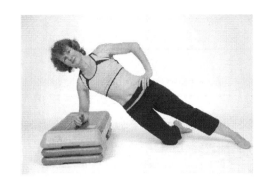

» Lean into your forearm as you straighten your top (opposite) leg.

» Push through your top foot to move your bottom knee away from the chair.

» Lower your hips.

» Endeavour to keep your body in a straight line and your head in line with your body.

» Hold.

» Switch sides.

BEGINNER SIDE PLANK 6—45 DEGREES

FOREARM ON 1ST OR 2ND STEP, RESTING ON SIDE OF KNEE (LOWER LEG), BOTH KNEES BENT

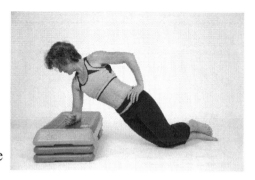

» Kneel at a 45 degree angle away from a step.

» Place one forearm on the step with your shoulder directly over your elbow.

» Lean into your forearm as you straighten your top (opposite) leg.

» Push through your top foot to move your bottom knee away from the step.

» Bend your top knee and rest your thighs together.

» Lower your hips.

» Endeavour to keep your body in a straight line and your head in line with your body.

» Hold.

» Switch sides.

Safety Recommendation:

» If you are not accustomed to bearing weight through one arm, consider keeping the other hand on the step for additional support until you build more shoulder strength.

BEGINNER SIDE PLANK 6—90 DEGREES

FOREARM ON 1ST OR 2ND STEP, RESTING ON SIDE OF KNEE (LOWER LEG), BOTH KNEES BENT

» Kneel sideways from a step.

» Place one forearm on the step with your shoulder directly over your elbow.

» Lean into your forearm as you straighten your top (opposite) leg.

» Push through your top foot to move your bottom knee away from the chair.

» Bend your top knee and rest your thighs together.

» Lower your hips.

» Endeavour to keep your body in a straight line and your head in line with your body.

» Hold.

» Switch sides.

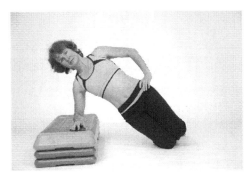

Safety Recommendation:

» If you are not accustomed to bearing weight through one arm, consider supporting your shoulder joint with the other hand until you build more shoulder strength.

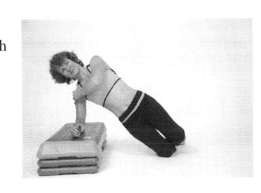

THE BEGINNER ROLL

The "Roll" teaches your body to be able to move in and out of positions with your natural abdominal brace in place.

The Roll is an exercise in which you transition as a block, with perfect form, between Side Planks and Planks. During the "Roll", support is transferred from one hand or forearm to the other while keeping your torso aligned.

Contract your abdominals the entire time as you transition from the Side Plank on your right at 90 degrees, to a Side Plank (still on your right) at 45 degrees, to a Plank into a Side Plank on your left at 45 degrees, and eventually into a Side Plank on your left at 90 degrees.

Photos on the right illustrate a Beginner level roll which can be done with any other combination of the Plank and Side Plank.

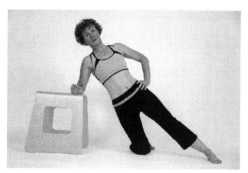
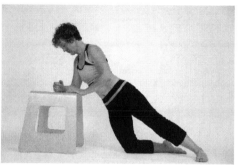
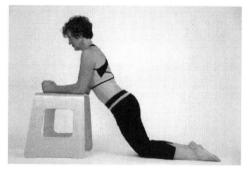
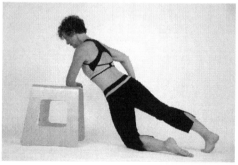
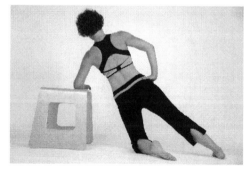

7. Active Plank Poses

Planks are always easier than Side Planks and should be explored first. The Active level Planks are appropriate for individuals who are currently participating in a regular exercise program and capable of doing all their own housework.

I encourage you to ensure that all foundational elements in Chapter 3 are considered prior to exploring these exercises. That chapter covers your breath, posture, and abdominal musculature—all essential elements to supporting your pose.

Hold times, repetitions, and training frequency are covered in Chapter 4—Frequently Asked Questions.

You may even run through the Beginner level Planks as a warmup to the ones we are going to explore next.

As you enter into every Plank, you should set your shoulders by gently drawing your shoulder blades downward and toward each other.

ACTIVE PLANK 1

HANDS ON FLOOR, RESTING ON KNEES

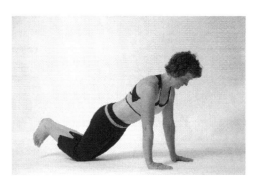

- » Kneel on your hands and knees with your shoulders directly over your hands.

- » Keep you hands shoulder-width apart.

- » Lean into your hands as you move your knees back.

- » Lower your hips.

- » Endeavour to keep your body in a straight line and your head in line with your body.

- » Hold.

Safety Recommendation:

- » If you have had low back pain in the past, keep your hips raised slightly towards the ceiling. Once you have mastered this level without any strain on your back, drop your hips and bring them in line with your body.

ACTIVE PLANK 2

FOREARMS ON FLOOR, RESTING ON KNEES

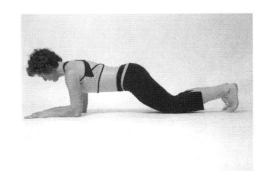

» Kneel on your forearms and knees with your shoulders directly over your elbows.

» Keep you forearms shoulder-width apart.

» Lean into your forearms as you move your knees back.

» Lower your hips.

» Endeavour to keep your body in a straight line and your head in line with your body.

» Hold.

Safety Recommendation:

» If you have had low back pain in the past, keep your hips raised slightly towards the ceiling. Once you have mastered this level without any strain on your back, drop your hips and bring them in line with your body.

ACTIVE PLANK 3

HANDS ON CHAIR, RESTING ON FEET

» Bend from your hips.

» Place your hands on a chair with your shoulders directly over your hands.

» Keep your hands shoulder-width apart.

» Lean into your hands as you step back with your feet hip-width apart.

» Lower your hips.

» Endeavour to keep your body in a straight line and your head in line with your body.

» Hold.

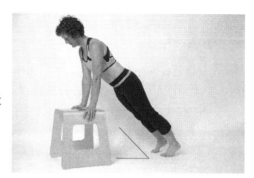

Safety Recommendation:

» If you have had low back pain in the past, keep your hips raised slightly towards the ceiling. Once you have mastered this level without any strain on your back, drop your hips and bring them in line with your body.

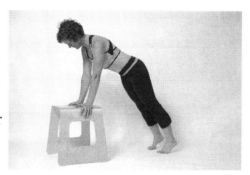

Challenging Variation 1:

» Follow the above steps but place your hands on a step stool or the first step in a stairwell.

Challenging Variation 2:

» Transfer weight from one foot to the other foot. (Weight transfer should be practiced before actually lifting a leg.)

» When you are able to lift one foot, hold for 3 to 5 seconds and then slowly transfer your weight to the other foot.

ACTIVE PLANK 4

FOREARMS ON CHAIR, RESTING ON FEET

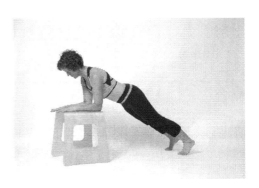

» Bend from your hips.

» Place your forearms on a chair with your shoulders directly over your elbows.

» Keep your forearms shoulder-width apart.

» Lean into your forearms as you step back with your feet hip-width apart.

» Lower your hips.

» Endeavour to keep your body in a straight line and your head in line with your body.

» Hold.

Safety Recommendation:

» If you have had low back pain in the past, keep your hips raised slightly towards the ceiling. Once you have mastered this level without any strain on your back, drop your hips and bring them in line with your body.

Challenging Variation:

» Follow the above steps but place your forearms on a step stool or the first step in a stairwell.

ACTIVE PLANK 5

HANDS ON BALL, BALL RESTING AGAINST SOFA, FEET ON FLOOR

» Bend from your hips.

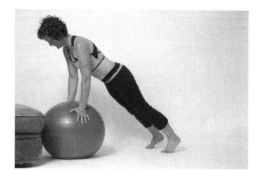

» Place your hands on a burst resistant ball (resting against a sofa) with your shoulders directly over your hands.

» Place your hands shoulder-width apart at an equal distance from the center of the ball.

» Lean into your hands as you step back with your feet hip-width apart.

» Lower your hips.

» Endeavour to keep your body in a straight line and your head in line with your body.

» Hold.

Challenging Variation:

» Place the ball an inch or so away from the sofa or solid chair. This will allow you to increase the multidirectional challenge for your arms and torso—with back up support if need be.

ACTIVE PLANK 6

HANDS ON BALL, FEET ON FLOOR

» Bend from your hips.

» Place your hands on a burst resistant ball with your shoulders directly over your hands.

» Place your hands shoulder-width apart at an equal distance from the center of the ball.

» Lean into your hands as you step back with your feet hip-width apart.

» Lower your hips.

» Endeavour to keep your body in a straight line and your head in line with your body.

» Hold.

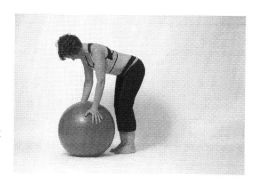

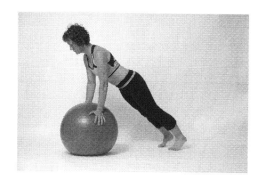

ACTIVE PLANK 7

HANDS ON BALL, FEET ON FLOOR, MOVING BALL IN A CONTROLLED MANNER

» Bend from your hips.

» Place your hands on a burst resistant ball with your shoulders directly over your hands.

» Place your hands shoulder-width apart at an equal distance from the center of the ball.

» Lean into your hands as you step back with your feet hip-width apart.

» Lower your hips.

» Endeavour to keep your body in a straight line and your head in line with your body.

» Move the ball in a controlled manner 2 inches to the right and then 2 inches to the left.

» Move the ball in a controlled manner 2 inches forward and then 2 inches back.

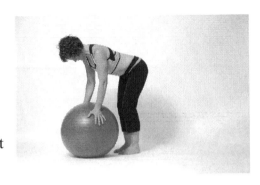

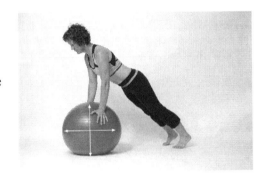

ACTIVE PLANK 8

HANDS ON FLOOR, LOWER THIGHS RESTING ON BALL

» Kneel tall behind a burst resistant ball. The ideal ball size is one in which your thighs are parallel to the floor when you are sitting on it.

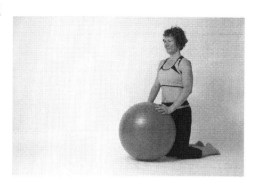

» Lower yourself onto the ball and press your hands firmly and evenly into the floor.

» Walk out on your hands until the ball rests under your lower thighs.

» Tighten your abdominals as soon as your pelvis leaves the ball so as not to have your low back sag towards the floor.

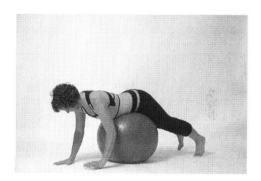

» Endeavour to keep your body in a straight line and your head in line with your body.

» Hold.

» Carefully walk your hands back to your start position.

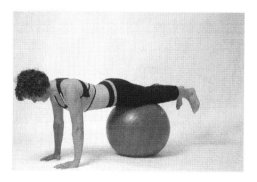

Challenging Variation:

» Transfer your weight onto one thigh, lifting the other thigh an inch or so off the ball.

» Hold for 2 to 3 seconds, alternating sides 2 to 5 times.

ACTIVE PLANK 9

HANDS ON FLOOR, LOWER LEGS RESTING ON BALL

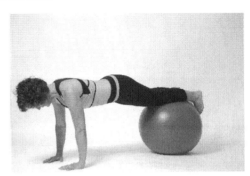

» Kneel tall behind a burst resistant ball. The ideal ball size is one in which your thighs are parallel to the floor when you are sitting on it.

» Lower yourself onto the ball and press your hands firmly and evenly into the floor.

» Walk out on your hands until the ball rests under your lower legs.

» Tighten your abdominals as soon as your pelvis leaves the ball so as not to have your low back sag towards the floor.

» Endeavour to keep your body in a straight line and your head in line with your body.

» Hold.

» Carefully walk your hands back to your start position.

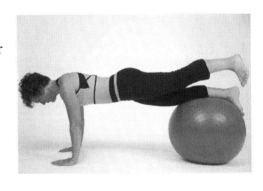

Challenging Variation:

» Transfer your weight onto one shin and lift the other leg an inch or so off the ball.

» Hold for 2 to 3 seconds, alternating sides 2 to 5 times.

ACTIVE PLANK 10

HANDS ON BALL, FEET RESTING ON FLOOR, MOVING BALL CLOCKWISE/ COUNTERCLOCKWISE

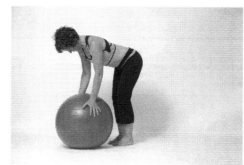

» Bend from your hips.

» Place your hands on a burst resistant ball with your shoulders directly over your hands.

» Place your hands shoulder-width apart at an equal distance from the center of the ball.

» Lean into your hands as you step back with your feet hip-width apart.

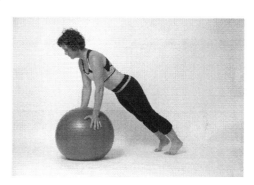

» Lower your hips.

» Endeavour to keep your body in a straight line and your head in line with your body.

» Move the ball in a controlled manner clockwise and counterclockwise (within a 2 to 6 inch range) for the duration of your hold.

8. Active Side Plank Poses

Side Planks are always more challenging than Planks. They require more strength through the shoulder, elbow, and wrist on the supporting side. They also require more strength through the lateral musculature of the torso, hips, and ankles.

The Active level Side Planks are appropriate for individuals who are currently participating in a regular exercise program and capable of doing all their own housework.

I encourage you to explore the Plank poses first to allow you to estimate the intensity of your Side Plank.

The Side Planks are labelled either Side Plank (number)—45 Degrees or Side Plank (number)—90 Degrees. A Side Plank (number)—45 Degrees identifies the position as midway between a Plank and a Side Plank (number)—90 Degrees.

As you enter into every Side Plank, you should set your shoulders by gently drawing your shoulder blades downward and toward each other.

In addition, while performing the Side Plank, the free hand can either rest on the surface or over the supporting shoulder.

ACTIVE SIDE PLANK 1—45 DEGREES

HAND ON CHAIR, FEET ON FLOOR

» Stand at a 45 degree angle from a chair.

» Bend from your hips.

» Place one hand on the center of the chair. Keep your shoulder directly over your hand.

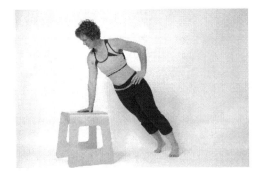

» Lean into your hand.

» Step away from the chair.

» Keep your feet parallel to one another at a 45 degree angle to the chair.

» Lower your hips.

» Endeavour to keep your body in a straight line and your head in line with your body.

» Hold.

» Switch sides.

Safety Recommendation:

» If you are not used to bearing weight on one arm, consider keeping the other hand on the chair or step for additional support until you build more shoulder strength.

Challenging Variation:

» Follow the above steps but place your hand on a lower surface, such as the second or first step in a stairwell. The lower the height, the more intense the load on your shoulder and your core.

ACTIVE SIDE PLANK 1—90 DEGREES

HAND ON A CHAIR, FEET ON FLOOR

» Stand sideways to a chair.

» Bend from your hips.

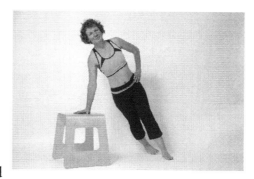

» Place one hand on the center of the chair. Keep your shoulder directly over your hand.

» Lean into your hand.

» Step away from the chair.

» Keep your feet parallel to the chair. When your right hand is supporting you, your left foot will be the lead foot and vice versa.

» Lower your hips.

» Endeavour to keep your body in a straight line and your head in line with your body.

» Hold.

» Switch sides.

Challenging Variation:

» Follow the above steps but place your hand on a lower surface such as the second or first step in a stairwell. The lower the height, the more intense the load on your shoulder and your core.

ACTIVE SIDE PLANK 2—45 DEGREES

HAND ON FLOOR, RESTING ON KNEE, ONE KNEE BENT

» Sit sideways on the floor.

» Place one hand on the floor directly beneath your shoulder.

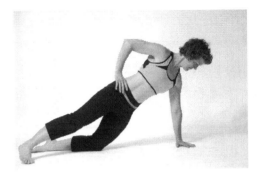

» Slide your knees back so that your thighs are in line with your body.

» Straighten your top (opposite) leg.

» Keep your bottom knee bent.

» Raise your hips.

» Push through your top foot to allow you to move your bottom knee away from your hand.

» Rotate your legs and body 45 degrees towards the floor.

» Endeavour to keep your body in a straight line and your head in line with your body.

» Hold.

» Switch sides.

Safety Recommendation:

» If you are not used to bearing weight on one arm, consider keeping the other hand on the floor for additional support until you build more shoulder strength.

ACTIVE SIDE PLANK 2—90 DEGREES

HAND ON FLOOR, RESTING ON KNEE, ONE KNEE BENT

» Sit sideways on the floor.

» Place one hand on the floor directly beneath your shoulder.

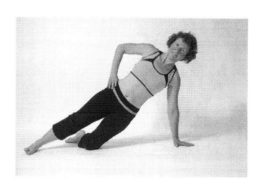

» Slide your knees back so that your thighs are in line with your body.

» Straighten your top (opposite) leg.

» Keep your bottom knee bent.

» Raise your hips.

» Push through your top foot to allow you to move your bottom knee away from your hand.

» Endeavour to keep your body in a straight line and your head in line with your body.

» Hold.

» Switch sides.

Safety Recommendation:

» If you are not used to putting weight through one arm, consider supporting your shoulder joint with the other hand until you build more shoulder strength.

Challenging Variation:

» Follow the above steps and once in the pose, raise and lower your top leg 2 to 3 inches, leading with your heel.

» Repeat for the duration of your hold.

ACTIVE SIDE PLANK 3—45 DEGREES

HAND ON FLOOR, RESTING ON SIDE OF KNEE

» Sit sideways on the floor.

» Place one hand on the floor directly beneath your shoulder.

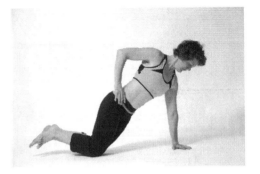

» Slide your knees back so that your thighs are in line with your body.

» Keep both knees bent.

» Raise your hips.

» Rotate your legs and body 45 degrees towards the floor.

» Endeavour to keep your body in a straight line and your head in line with your body.

» Hold.

» Switch sides.

Safety Recommendation:

» If you are not used to putting weight through one arm, consider keeping the other hand on the floor for additional support until you build more shoulder strength.

ACTIVE SIDE PLANK 3—90 DEGREES

HAND ON FLOOR, RESTING ON SIDE OF KNEE (LOWER LEG)

» Sit sideways on the floor.

» Place one hand on the floor directly beneath your shoulder.

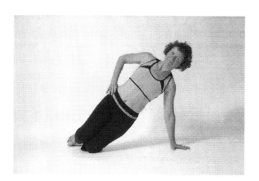

» Slide your knees back so that your thighs are in line with your body.

» Keep both knees bent.

» Raise your hips.

» Endeavour to keep your body in a straight line and your head in line with your body.

» Hold.

» Switch sides.

Safety Recommendation:

» If you are not used to bearing weight on one arm, consider supporting your shoulder joint with the other hand until you build more shoulder strength.

ACTIVE SIDE PLANK 4—45 DEGREES

FOREARM ON CHAIR, FEET ON FLOOR

» Stand at a 45 degree angle from a chair.

» Bend from your hips.

» Place one forearm on the center of the chair. Keep your shoulder directly over your elbow.

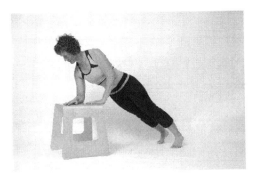

» Lean into your forearm.

» Step away from the chair as indicated in the photo.

» Keep your feet parallel to one another at a 45 degree angle to the chair.

» Lower your hips.

» Endeavour to keep your body in a straight line and your head in line with your body.

» Hold.

» Switch sides.

Safety Recommendation:

» If you are not used to bearing weight on one arm, consider keeping the other hand on the chair (as shown in the picture) for additional support until you build more shoulder strength.

Challenging Variation:

» Follow the above steps but place your forearm on a lower surface such as the second or first step in a stairwell. The lower the height, the more intense the load on your shoulder and your core.

ACTIVE SIDE PLANK 4—90 DEGREES

FOREARM ON CHAIR, FEET ON FLOOR

» Stand sideways to a chair.

» Bend from your hips.

» Place one forearm on the center of the chair. Keep your shoulder directly over your elbow.

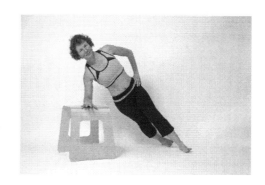

» Lean into your forearm.

» Step away from the chair as indicated in the photo.

» Keep your feet parallel to the chair.

» When your right hand is supporting you, your left foot will be the lead foot and vice versa.

» Lower your hips.

» Endeavour to keep your body in a straight line and your head in line with your body.

» Hold.

» Switch sides.

Challenging Variation:

» Follow the above steps but place your forearm on a lower surface such as the second or first step in a stairwell. The lower the height, the more intense the load on your shoulder and your core.

ACTIVE SIDE PLANK 5—45 DEGREES
FOREARM ON FLOOR, RESTING ON KNEE, TOP KNEE STRAIGHT

» Lie on your side on the floor.

» Place one forearm on the floor with your elbow in from your shoulder.

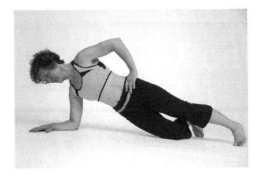

» Slide your knees back so that your thighs are in line with your body.

» Straighten your top (opposite) leg.

» Bend your bottom knee.

» Raise your hips. Your shoulder will align over your elbow.

» Rotate your body and legs 45 degrees to the floor.

» Endeavour to keep your body in a straight line and your head in line with your body.

» Hold.

» Switch sides.

ACTIVE SIDE PLANK 5—90 DEGREES

FOREARM ON FLOOR, RESTING ON KNEE, TOP KNEE STRAIGHT

» Lie on your side on the floor.

» Place one forearm on the floor with your elbow in from your shoulder.

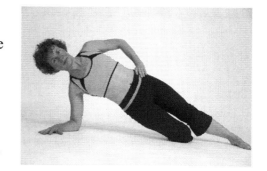

» Slide your knees back so that your thighs are in line with your body.

» Straighten your top (opposite) leg.

» Bend your bottom knee.

» Raise your hips. Your shoulder will align over your elbow.

» Endeavour to keep your body in a straight line and your head in line with your body.

» Hold.

» Switch sides.

Safety Recommendation:

» If you are not used to bearing weight on one arm, consider supporting your shoulder joint with the other hand until you build more shoulder strength.

Challenging Variation:

» Raise and lower your top leg 4 to 6 inches, leading with your heel.

» Repeat for the duration of your hold.

ACTIVE SIDE PLANK 6—45 DEGREES

FOREARM ON FLOOR, RESTING ON SIDE OF KNEE

» Lie on your side on the floor.

» Place one forearm on the floor with your elbow in from your shoulder.

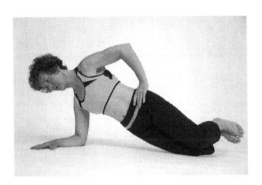

» Slide your knees back so that your thighs are in line with your body.

» Bend both knees.

» Raise your hips. Your shoulder will align over your shoulder.

» Rotate your body and legs 45 degrees to the floor.

» Endeavour to keep your body in a straight line and your head in line with your body.

» Hold.

» Switch sides.

Safety Recommendation:

» If you are not used to putting weight through one forearm, consider keeping the other hand on the floor for additional support until you build more shoulder strength.

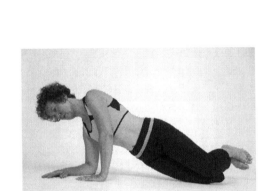

ACTIVE SIDE PLANK 6—90 DEGREES

FOREARM ON FLOOR, RESTING ON SIDE OF KNEE (LOWER LEG)

» Lie on your side on the floor.

» Place one forearm on the floor with your elbow in from your shoulder.

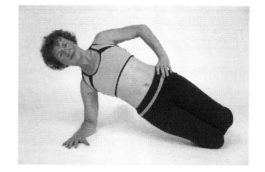

» Slide your knees back so that your thighs are in line with your body.

» Bend both knees.

» Raise your hips. Your shoulder will align over your elbow.

» Endeavour to keep your body in a straight line and your head in line with your body.

» Hold.

» Switch sides.

Safety Recommendation:

» If you are not used to bearing weight on one forearm, consider supporting your shoulder joint with the other hand until you build more shoulder strength.

THE ACTIVE ROLL

Active level individuals will benefit from the "Roll" mentioned in the book, *The Ultimate Back Fitness and Performance,* by Dr. Stuart McGill. The Roll is an exercise where you transition as a block, with perfect form, between Side Planks and Planks. During the "Roll", support is transferred from one hand or forearm to the other while keeping your torso aligned.

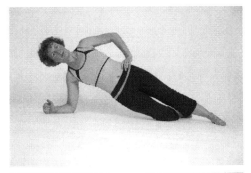

Contract your abdominals the entire time as you transition from the Side Plank on your right at 90 degrees, to a Side Plank (still on your right) at 45 degrees, to a Plank into a Side Plank on your left at 45 degrees, and eventually into a Side Plank on your left at 90 degrees.

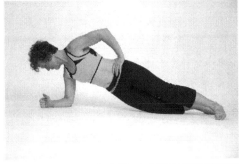

It has been my experience that individuals performing Active level Planks and Side Planks learn to do the "Roll" best if they first do so with Beginner Side Planks. The concept of bracing the abdominals and moving your body as a solid "Plank" is one that is both challenging and fun!

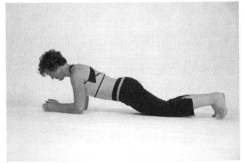

The "Roll" teaches your body to be able to move in and out of positions with the abdominal brace in place.

Photos on the right illustrate an Active level roll which can be done with any other combination of the Plank and Side Plank.

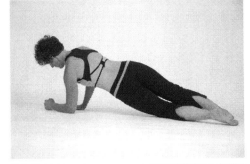

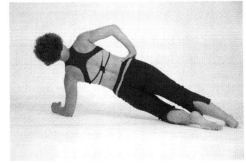

9. Athletic Plank Poses

Planks are always easier than Side Planks and should be explored first. Athletic level Planks are appropriate for individuals who have been involved in a regular exercise program for at least a year (three or four exercise sessions per week), who have started to incorporate an exercise ball, or are not intimidated by the thought of an exercise ball as part of their exercise routine.

I encourage you to ensure that all foundational elements in Chapter 3 are considered prior to exploring the exercises. That chapter covers breath, posture, and abdominal musculature—all essential elements to supporting your exercise.

Hold times, repetitions, training frequency are covered in Chapter 4—Frequently Asked Questions.

You may even run through the Active level Planks as a warmup to the ones we are going to explore next.

Athletic level individuals will benefit from the following drill (found in *Ultimate Back Fitness and Performance* by Dr. Stuart McGill) to train their body to be stable while breathing hard:

1. Perform an intensive cardiovascular exercise such as stationary bike, treadmill run, or sprint at an intensity that causes you to breathe hard.

2. Immediately stop and perform your Plank pose.

Note that you should start your Plank at a level that is less intense than you would with normal breathing.

As you enter into every Plank, you should set your shoulders by gently drawing your shoulder blades downward and toward each other.

ATHLETIC PLANK 1

FOREARMS ON BALL, BALL ON FLOOR, FEET ON FLOOR

» Kneel behind a burst resistant exercise ball on the floor.

» Bend from the hips and place your forearms shoulder-width apart at an equal distance from the center of the ball.

» Lean into your forearms.

» Step back and place your feet hip-width apart and parallel to one another.

» Endeavour to keep your body in a straight line and your head in line with your body.

» Hold.

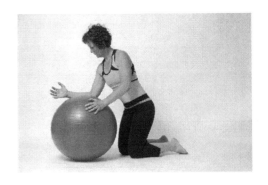

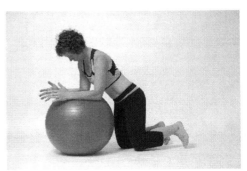

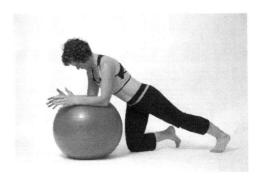

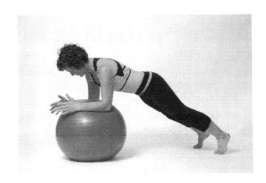

ATHLETIC PLANK 2

FOREARMS ON BALL, BALL ON FLOOR, FEET ON FLOOR, MOVING BALL IN A CONTROLLED MANNER

» Kneel behind a burst resistant exercise ball on the floor.

» Bend from the hips and place your forearms shoulder-width apart at an equal distance from the center of the ball.

» Lean into your forearms

» Step back and place your feet hip-width apart and parallel to one another.

» Endeavour to keep your body in a straight line and your head in line with your body.

» Move the ball in a controlled manner 2 inches to the right and then 2 inches to the left.

» Move the ball in a controlled manner 2 inches forward and then 2 inches back.

» Move the ball in a controlled manner on a diagonal pattern as indicated in the bottom photo (where the **up** arrow represents a movement to the model's right and the **down** arrow represents a move to the model's left.)

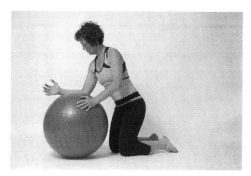

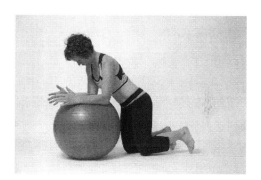

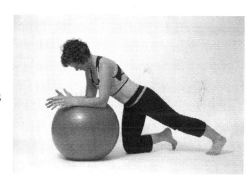

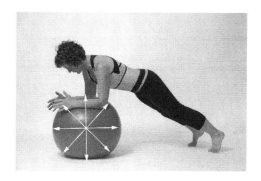

ATHLETIC PLANK 3

FOREARMS ON BALL, BALL ON FLOOR, FEET ON FLOOR, MOVING BALL IN CONTROLLED MANNER

» Kneel behind a burst resistant exercise ball.

» Bend from the hips and place your forearms shoulder-width apart at an equal distance from the center of the ball.

» Lean into your forearms.

» Step back and place your feet hip-width apart and parallel to one another.

» Endeavour to keep your body in a straight line and your head in line with your body.

» Move the ball through an imaginary maze, starting with a 2 inch diameter circle gradually building to a 6 inch diameter circle clockwise, returning counterclockwise.

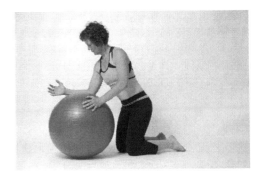

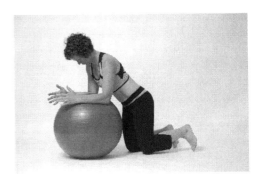

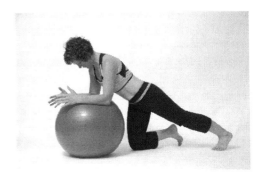

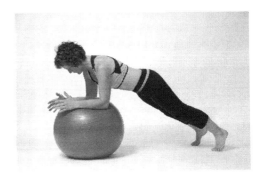

ATHLETIC PLANK 4

FOREARMS ON BALL, BALL ON FLOOR, FEET ON FLOOR, TRANSFER WEIGHT TO ONE FOOT

» Kneel behind a burst resistant exercise ball.

» Place your forearms shoulder-width apart at an equal distance from the center of the ball.

» Lean into your forearms.

» Step back and place your feet hip-width apart and parallel to one another.

» Transfer your weight to one foot and lift the other several inches from the floor. Hold for 3 to 5 seconds and then slowly transfer your weight to the other foot.

» Endeavour to keep your body in a straight line and your head in line with your body.

» Repeat back and forth until your hold time is completed.

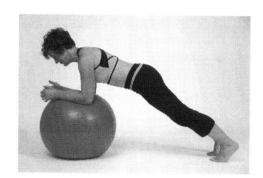

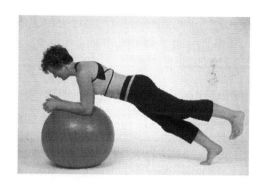

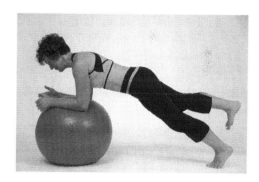

ATHLETIC PLANK 5

HANDS AND FEET ON FLOOR

» Start on your hands and knees.

» Place your hands beneath your shoulders.

» Lean into your hands.

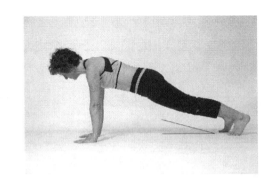

» Step back and place your feet hip-width apart and parallel to one another.

» Lower your hips.

» Endeavour to keep your body in a straight line and your head in line with your body.

Challenging Variation #1:

» Follow the above steps but this time place one hand on a medicine ball while the other rests on floor.

Challenging Variation #2:

» Follow the above steps but this time place both hands on a single medicine ball.

Challenging Variation #3:

» Follow the above steps but this time place each hand on a separate medicine ball.

ATHLETIC PLANK 6

HANDS AND ONE FOOT ON FLOOR

» Place your hands on the floor shoulder-width apart.

» Lean into your hands.

» Step back and place your feet hip-width apart and parallel to one another.

» Transfer your weight to one foot and lift the other several inches from the floor. Hold for 3 to 5 seconds and then slowly transfer your weight to the other foot.

» Endeavour to keep your body in a straight line and your head in line with your body.

» Repeat back and forth until your hold time is completed.

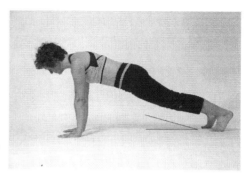

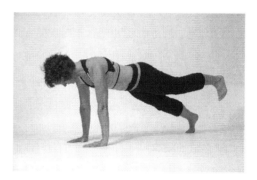

ATHLETIC PLANK 7

FOREARMS AND FEET ON FLOOR

» Place your forearms on the floor shoulder-width apart.

» Lean into your forearms.

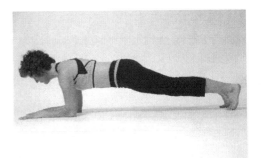

» Step back and place your feet close together and parallel to one another.

» Endeavour to keep your body in a straight line and your head in line with your body.

» Hold.

Challenging Variation:

» Follow the above steps, transfer weight to one foot and lift the other foot several inches from floor.

» Repeat back and forth until your hold time is completed.

ATHLETIC PLANK 8

HANDS ON FLOOR, FEET ON BALL

» Kneel tall behind a burst resistant ball. The ideal ball size is one in which your thighs are parallel to the floor when you are sitting on it.

» Lower yourself onto the ball and press your hands firmly and evenly into the floor.

» Walk your hands out until the ball rests under your feet.

» Hold.

» Walk your hands back to your start position or bring your feet to the floor.

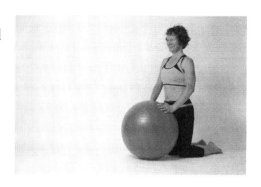
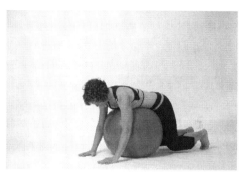
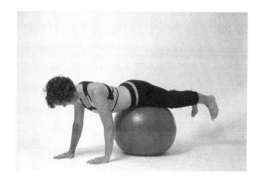
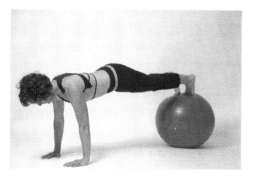

ATHLETIC PLANK 9

HANDS ON FLOOR, LEGS ON BALL, ALTERNATING LEG LIFTS

» Kneel tall behind a burst resistant ball. The ideal ball size is one in which your thighs are parallel to the floor when you are sitting on it.

» Lower yourself onto the ball and press your hands firmly and evenly into the floor.

» Walk your hands out until the ball rests under your shins.

» Transfer your weight onto one thigh and lift the other thigh off the ball.

» Hold for 2 to 3 seconds alternating sides 2 to 5 times.

» Walk your hands back to your start position or bring your feet to the floor.

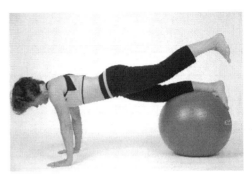

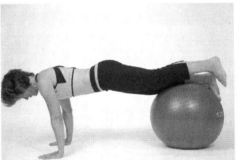

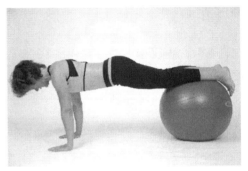

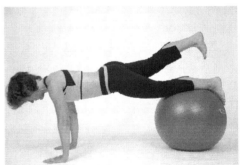

ATHLETIC PLANK 10

HANDS ON BALL, FEET ON BENCH

» Bend from the waist and place your hands shoulder-width apart at an equal distance from the center of a burst resistant exercise ball.

» Lean into your hands.

» Step back and place your feet onto a bench or chair—feet hip-width apart and parallel to one another.

» Endeavour to keep your body in a straight line and your head in line with your body.

» Hold.

Gentler Variation:

» Follow the above steps but this time step back onto a lower surface.

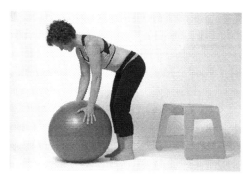

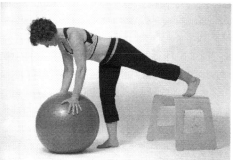

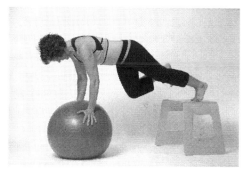

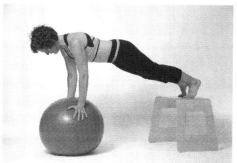

10. Athletic Side Plank Poses

Side Planks are always more challenging than planks. They require more strength through the shoulder, elbow, and wrist on the supporting side. They also require more strength through the lateral musculature of the torso, hips, and ankles.

The Athletic level Side Planks are appropriate for individuals involved in a regular exercise program (three or four exercise sessions per week) that includes upper body strength training.

I encourage you to explore the Plank poses first to allow you to estimate the intensity of your Side Plank.

Athletic level individuals will benefit from the following drill (found in *Ultimate Back Fitness and Performance* by Dr. Stuart McGill) to train their body to be stable while breathing hard:

1.   Perform an intensive cardiovascular exercise such as stationary bike, treadmill run, or sprint at an intensity that causes you to breath hard.

2.   Immediately stop and perform your Side Plank pose.

Note that you should start your Side Plank at a level that is less intense than you would with normal breathing.

As you enter into every Side Plank, you should set your shoulders by gently drawing your shoulder blades downward and toward each other.

In addition, while performing the Side Plank, the free hand can either rest on the surface or over the supporting shoulder.

ATHLETIC SIDE PLANK 1—45 DEGREES

FOREARM ON BALL, BALL ON FLOOR, FEET ON FLOOR

» Stand at a 45 degree angle from a ball.

» Bend from your hips.

» Place one forearm on the center of the ball. Keep
your shoulder directly over your elbow.

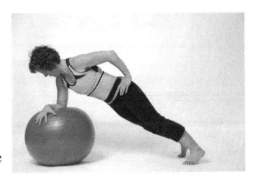

» Lean into your forearm.

» Step away from the ball.

» Keep your feet parallel to one another at a 45 degree
angle to the ball.

» Lower your hips.

» Endeavour to keep your body in a straight line and your head in line with your body.

» Hold.

» Switch sides.

Safety Recommendation:

» Putting weight through one arm on an unstable surface is harder than it looks. Consider
keeping the other hand on the ball for additional support until you build more shoulder
strength.

ATHLETIC SIDE PLANK 1—90 DEGREES

FOREARM ON BALL, BALL ON FLOOR, FEET ON FLOOR

» Stand sideways to a ball.

» Bend from your hips.

» Place one forearm on the center of the ball. Keep your shoulder directly over your elbow.

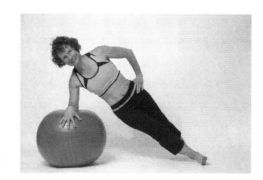

» Lean into your forearm.

» Step away from the ball.

» Keep your feet parallel to the ball. When your right hand is supporting you, your left foot will be the lead foot and vice versa.

» Lower your hips.

» Endeavour to keep your body in a straight line and your head in line with your body.

» Hold.

» Switch sides.

ATHLETIC SIDE PLANK 2—45 DEGREES

FOREARM ON FLOOR, RESTING ON FEET

» Rest your forearm on the floor with the elbow slightly in from the shoulder, your body and feet rotated 45 degrees away from center line.

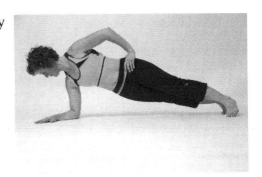

» Lean into your forearm.

» Raise your hips.

» Rest on your toes.

» Endeavour to keep your body in a straight line and your head in line with your body.

» Hold.

» Switch sides.

ATHLETIC SIDE PLANK 2—90 DEGREES

FOREARM ON FLOOR, RESTING ON FEET

» Rest your forearm on the floor with the elbow slightly in from the shoulder and your body facing the front.

» Lean into your forearm.

» Raise your hips.

» Rest on your outer edge of bottom foot.

» Endeavour to keep your body in a straight line and your head in line with your body.

» Hold.

» Switch sides.

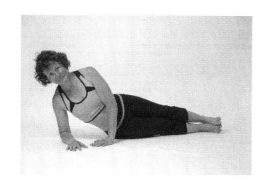

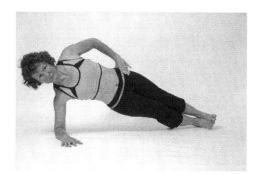

Challenging Variation:

» Follow the above steps. Once in the pose, raise and lower your top leg, leading with your heel.

» Repeat for the duration of your hold.

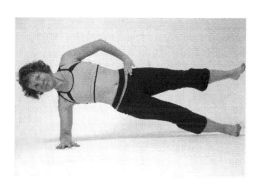

ATHLETIC SIDE PLANK 3—45 DEGREES

HAND ON FLOOR, FEET ON BOSU

» Rest your hand on the floor with your hand slightly in from the shoulder and your body and feet rotated 45 degrees away from center line.

» Lean into your hand.

» Step onto the Bosu.

» Rest on your toes.

» Endeavour to keep your body in a straight line and your head in line with your body.

» Hold.

» Switch sides.

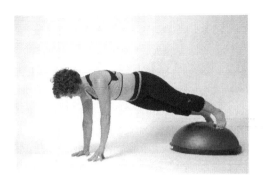

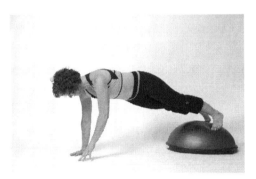

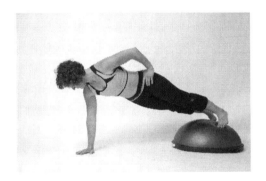

ATHLETIC SIDE PLANK 3—90 DEGREES

HAND ON FLOOR, FEET ON BOSU

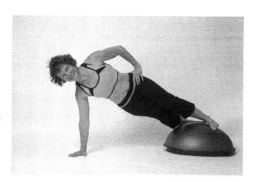

» Rest your hand on the floor with your hand slightly in from the shoulder, your body facing the front.

» Lean into your hand.

» Step onto the Bosu.

» Rest on the inside of your top foot and the outside of your bottom foot.

» Endeavour to keep your body in a straight line and your head in line with your body.

» Hold.

» Switch sides.

ATHLETIC SIDE PLANK 4—45 DEGREES

FOREARM ON FLOOR, LOWER LEGS ON BOSU

» Rest your forearm on the floor with your elbow slightly in from the shoulder, your body and feet rotated 45 degrees away from center line.

» Lean into your forearm.

» Step onto the Bosu.

» Rest on your toes.

» Endeavour to keep your body in a straight line and your head in line with your body.

» Hold.

» Switch sides.

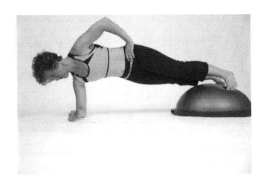

ATHLETIC SIDE PLANK 4—90 DEGREES

FOREARM ON FLOOR, LOWER LEGS ON BOSU

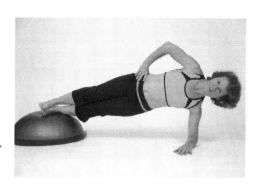

» Rest your forearm on the floor with your elbow slightly in from the shoulder, your body facing the front.

» Lean into your forearm.

» Step onto the Bosu.

» Rest on the inside of your top foot and the outside of your bottom foot.

» Endeavour to keep your body in a straight line and your head in line with your body.

» Hold.

» Switch sides.

ATHLETIC SIDE PLANK 5—90 DEGREES

FOREARM ON FLOOR, TOP FOOT ON FLOOR, BOTTOM LEG UP

» Rest your forearm on the floor with the elbow slightly in from the shoulder and your body facing the front.

» Lean into your forearm.

» Raise your hips.

» Rest on your inside edge of top foot.

» Bring bottom knee up towards your chest.

» Endeavour to keep your body in a straight line and your head in line with your body.

» Hold.

» Switch sides.

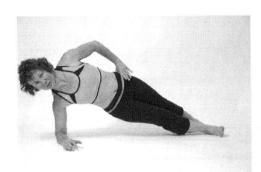

Variation:

» Rather than holding the bottom leg in a static position, slide the leg back touching your supporting foot with the heel of the bottom leg and back up towards your chest, repeating for the duration of your hold.

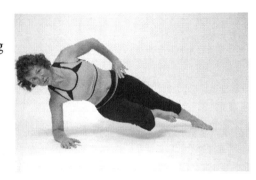

THE ATHLETIC ROLL

Athletic level individuals will benefit from the "Roll" mentioned in the book, *The Ultimate Back Fitness and Performance,* by Dr. Stuart McGill. The Roll is an exercise where you transition as a block, with perfect form, between Side Planks and Plank. During the "Roll", support is transferred from one hand or forearm to the other while keeping your torso aligned.

Contract your abdominals the entire time as you transition from the Side Plank on your right at 90 degrees, to a Side Plank (still on your right) at 45 degrees, to a Plank into a Side Plank on your left at 45 degrees, and eventually into a Side Plank on your left at 90 degrees.

The concept of bracing the abdominals and moving your body as a solid "Plank" is one that is both challenging and fun!

The "Roll" teaches your body to be able to move in and out of positions with the abdominal brace in place.

Photos on the right illustrate an Athletic level roll which can be done with any other combination of the Plank and Side Plank.

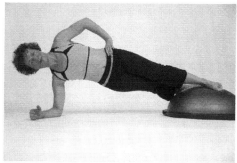

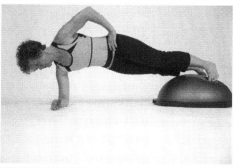

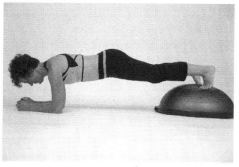

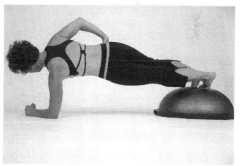

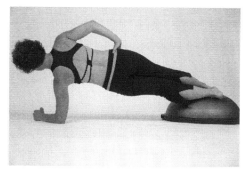

11. Elite Plank Poses

Planks are always easier than Side Planks and should be explored first. The Elite level Planks are, as the name implies, done by high level athletes. Elements of instability and progressive-loading are all involved.

There is not as much detail about how to get into the starting position for Elite level Planks as compared to the other levels. If you need more detail, please refer to the Active and Athletic level Planks which correspond to the appropriate Elite Plank poses.

I encourage you to ensure that all foundational elements in Chapter 3 are considered prior to exploring the poses. That chapter covers your breath, posture, and abdominal musculature—all essential elements to supporting your exercise. Hold times and frequency of training are covered in Chapter 4—Frequently Asked Questions. You may even run through the Athletic level Planks as a warmup to the ones we're going to explore next.

Elite level individuals will benefit from the following drill (found in *Ultimate Back Fitness and Performance* by Dr. Stuart McGill) to train their body to be stable while breathing hard:

1. Perform an intensive cardiovascular exercise such as stationary bike, treadmill run, or sprint at an intensity that causes you to breath hard.

2. Immediately stop and perform your Plank exercise.

Note that you should start your Plank at a level that is less intense than you would with normal breathing.

As you enter into every Plank, you should set your shoulders by gently drawing your shoulder blades downward and toward each other.

ELITE PLANK 1

THREE POINT SUPPORT FROM HANDS AND FEET

» Position yourself on your hands and feet. Keep hands close together and in line with your shoulders.

» Transfer weight onto your right hand.

» Raise your left arm until you can bring it in line with your body.

» Endeavour to keep your body in a straight line and your head in line with your body.

» Hold.

» Place your left hand on the floor and then lift your right arm while maintaining three point contact with the floor.

» Place your right hand on the floor and then lift your right leg while maintaining three point contact with the floor.

» Place your right foot on the floor and then lift your left leg while maintaining three point contact with the floor.

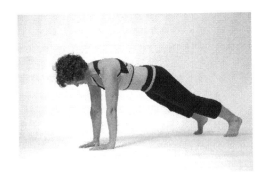

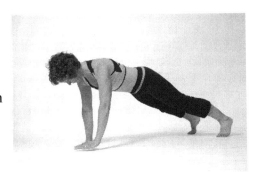

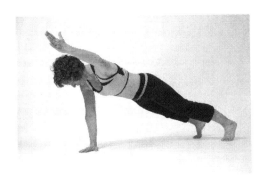

ELITE PLANK 2

THREE POINT SUPPORT FROM FEET AND FOREARMS

» Position yourself on your forearms and feet.

» Transfer weight onto your right forearm.

» Raise your left arm until you can bring it in line with your body.

» Endeavour to keep your body in a straight line and your head in line with your body.

» Hold.

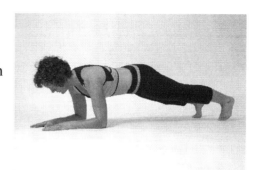

» Place your left forearm on the floor and then lift your right arm while maintaining three point contact with the floor.

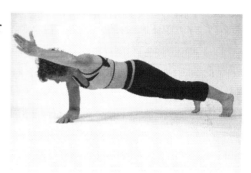

» Place your right forearm on the floor and then lift your right leg while maintaining three point contact with the floor.

» Place your right foot on the floor and then lift your left leg while maintaining three point contact with the floor.

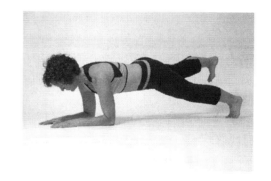

ELITE PLANK 3

TWO POINT SUPPORT, FOREARM AND FOOT

» Position yourself on your forearms and feet.

» Transfer weight onto your right forearm and left foot.

» Raise your left arm and right leg until you can bring them in line with your body.

» Endeavour to keep your body in a straight line and your head in line with your body.

» Hold.

» Place your left forearm and right foot back on the floor and repeat the above procedure using your right forearm and left leg.

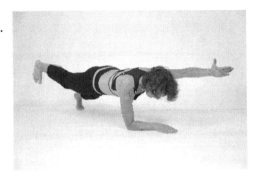

ELITE PLANK 4

TWO POINT SUPPORT FROM OPPOSITE HAND AND FOOT

» Position yourself on your hands and feet.

» Transfer weight onto your right hand and left foot.

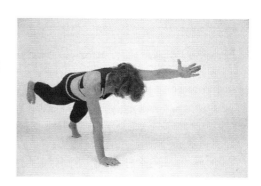

» Raise your left arm and right leg until you can bring them in line with your body.

» Endeavour to keep your body in a straight line and your head in line with your body.

» Hold.

» Place your left hand and right foot back on the floor and repeat the above procedure using your right arm and left leg.

ELITE PLANK 5

HANDS ON FLOOR, SINGLE FOOT ON BALL

» Start with your hands on the floor below your shoulders and your feet on a ball.

» Transfer your weight onto one foot and lift the other foot off the ball.

» Endeavour to keep your body in a straight line and your head in line with your body.

» Hold for 2 to 3 seconds and alternate sides.

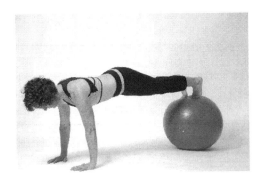

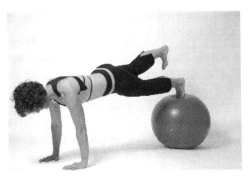

ELITE PLANK 6

HANDS ON A BALL WITH FOOT RAISED FROM STEP/CHAIR

» Start with your hands on a ball equal distance apart below your shoulders and your feet on a bench or chair.

» Transfer your weight onto one foot and lift the other foot off the ball.

» Endeavour to keep your body in a straight line and your head in line with your body.

» Hold for 2 to 3 seconds and alternate sides.

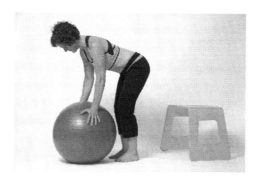

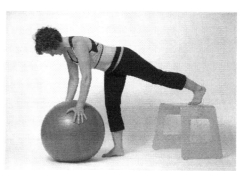

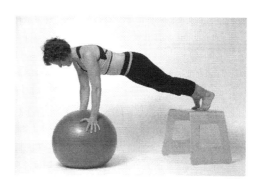

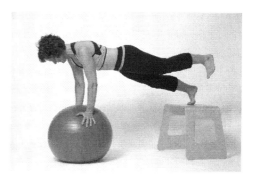

ELITE PLANK 7

FEET ON BALL, ONE HAND ON FLOOR

» Start with your hands on the floor below your breast bone and your feet on the ball.

» Transfer your weight onto one hand and lift the other arm gradually to the height of your body.

» Endeavour to keep your body in a straight line and your head in line with your body.

» Hold for 2 to 3 seconds and alternate sides.

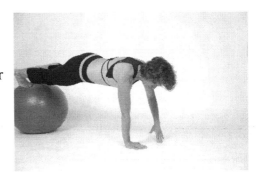

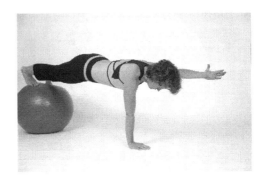

12. Elite Side Plank Poses

Side Planks are always more challenging than Planks. They require more strength through the shoulder, elbow, and wrist on the supporting side. They also require more strength through the lateral musculature of the torso, hips, and ankles.

The Elite level Side Planks are appropriate for individuals who have been involved in a regular exercise program (three or four exercise sessions per week) over several years that incorporates upper body strength training.

There is not as much detail about how to get into the starting position for Elite level Planks as compared to the other levels. If you need more detail, please refer to the Active and Athletic level Side Planks which correspond to the appropriate Elite Side Plank poses.

I encourage you to explore the Elite level Plank exercises first to allow you to estimate the intensity of your Side Plank.

Elite level individuals will benefit from the following drill (found in *Ultimate Back Fitness and Performance* by Dr. Stuart McGill) to train their body to be stable while breathing hard:

1.   Perform an intensive cardiovascular exercise such as stationary bike, treadmill run, or sprint at an intensity that causes you to breath hard.

2.   Immediately stop and perform your Side Plank pose.

Note that you should start your Side Plank at a level that is less intense than you would with normal breathing.

As you enter into every Side Plank, you should set your shoulders by gently drawing your shoulder blades downward and toward each other. In addition, while performing the Side Plank, the free hand can either rest on the surface or over the supporting shoulder.

ELITE SIDE PLANK 1—45 DEGREES

HAND ON FLOOR, LOWER FOOT ON BENCH

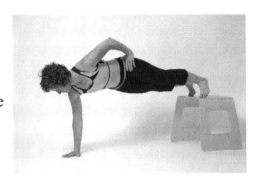

» Place your hand beneath your shoulder.

» Bring the balls of both feet onto the edge of a chair or bench.

» Rotate your body and feet 45 degrees away from the floor.

» Endeavour to keep your body in a straight line and your head in line with your body.

» Hold.

» Switch sides.

ELITE SIDE PLANK 1—90 DEGREES

HAND ON FLOOR, LOWER FOOT ON BENCH

» Place your right hand beneath your right shoulder.

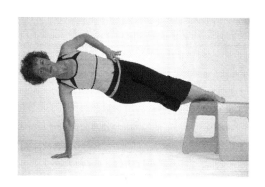

» Bring the outer edge of your bottom foot and the inner edge of your top foot onto the edge of a chair or bench.

» Endeavour to keep your body in a straight line and your head in line with your body.

» Hold.

» Switch sides.

ELITE SIDE PLANK 2

HAND ON FLOOR, LOWER FOOT ON BENCH, RAISE TOP LEG

» Rest on your right hand with your hand slightly in from your right shoulder.

» Bring the outer edge of your bottom foot onto the edge of a bench.

» Endeavour to keep your body in a straight line and your head in line with your body.

» Transfer weight onto both the outside of the bottom foot and your hand as you raise your top leg.

» Hold for 2 to 3 seconds.

» Repeat for the duration of your hold time.

» Switch sides.

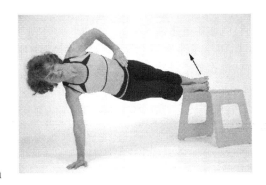

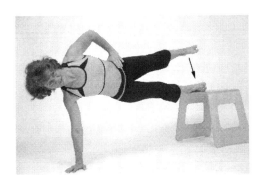

ELITE SIDE PLANK 3

FOREARM ON FLOOR, LOWER FOOT ON BENCH, RAISE TOP LEG

» Place your right elbow beneath your right shoulder.

» Rest through your entire forearm.

» Bring the outer edge of your bottom foot onto the edge of a bench.

» Raise your hips bringing your shoulder in line with your elbow.

» Endeavour to keep your body in a straight line and your head in line with your body.

» Transfer weight onto both the outside of the bottom foot and your forearm as you raise your top leg.

» Hold for 2 to 3 seconds.

» Repeat for the duration of your hold time.

» Switch sides.

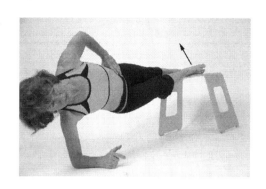

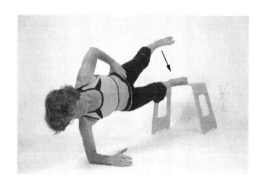

ELITE SIDE PLANK 4

HAND ON FLOOR, TOP FOOT ON BENCH, BEND AND STRAIGHTEN LOWER LEG

» Place your right hand beneath your right shoulder.

» Bring the inner edge of your top foot onto the edge of a bench.

» Raise your hips and bring your bottom foot under the bench.

» Bring your bottom knee towards your chest.

» Endeavour to keep your body in a straight line and your head in line with your body.

» Hold for 2 to 3 seconds.

» Repeat for duration of your hold time.

» Switch sides.

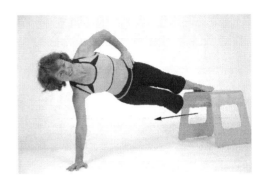

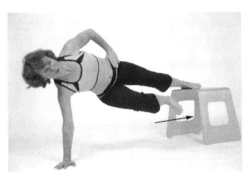

ELITE SIDE PLANK 5

FOREARM ON FLOOR, TOP FOOT ON BENCH, BEND AND STRAIGHTEN LOWER LEG

» Place your right elbow beneath your right shoulder.

» Rest through your entire forearm.

» Bring the inner edge of your top foot onto the edge of a bench.

» Raise your hips and bring your bottom foot under the bench.

» Endeavour to keep your body in a straight line and your head in line with your body.

» Repeat for duration of your hold time.

» Switch sides.

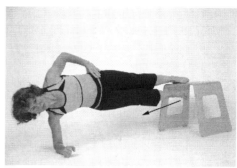

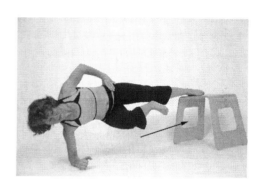

ELITE SIDE PLANK 6

HAND ON FLOOR, FEET RESTING ON CHAIR, LOWER AND RAISE PELVIS

» Place your right hand beneath your right shoulder.

» Bring the inner edge of your top foot and outer edge of the bottom foot onto the edge of a chair or bench.

» Drop your pelvis 4 to 6 inches below the line created between your bottom shoulder, hip, and feet.

» Return to start position.

» Repeat for duration of your hold time.

» Switch sides.

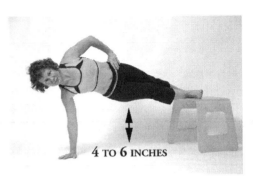

4 TO 6 INCHES

ELITE SIDE PLANK 7

FOREARM ON FLOOR, FEET RESTING ON BOSU, RAISE AND LOWER TOP LEG

» Rest on your forearm with your elbow slightly in from your shoulder.

» Bring the outer edge of your bottom foot onto the edge of a Bosu and bring your shoulder in line with your elbow.

» Transfer weight onto both the outside of the bottom foot and your forearm as you raise your top leg.

» Repeat for duration of your hold time.

» Endeavour to keep your body in a straight line and your head in line with your body.

» Switch sides.

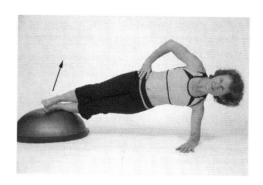

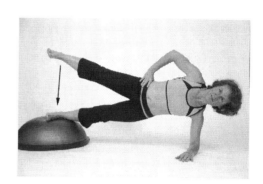

ELITE SIDE PLANK 8

HAND ON FLOOR, TOP FOOT RESTING ON BOSU, DRAW BOTTOM LEG UP TOWARDS CHEST

» Place your left hand beneath your left shoulder.

» Bring the inner edge of your top foot onto a Bosu.

» Transfer weight onto both the inside of the top foot and your hand as you bend your bottom hip and knee.

» Return your foot towards the Bosu.

» Repeat for the duration of your hold time.

» Endeavour to keep your body in a straight line and your head in line with your body.

» Switch sides.

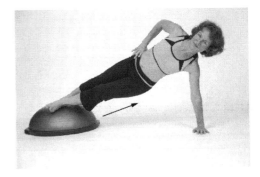

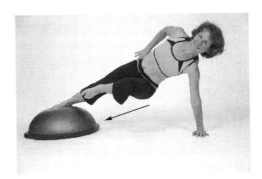

THE ELITE ROLL

Elite level individuals will benefit from the "Roll" mentioned in the book, *The Ultimate Back Fitness and Performance,* by Dr. Stuart McGill. The Roll is an exercise where you transition as a block, with perfect form, between Side Plank and Plank. During the "Roll", support is transferred from one hand or forearm to the other while keeping your torso aligned.

Contract your abdominals the entire time as you transition from the Side Plank on your right at 90 degrees, to a Side Plank (still on your right) at 45 degrees, to a Plank into a Side Plank on your left at 45 degrees, and eventually into a Side Plank on your left at 90 degrees.

The concept of bracing the abdominals and moving your body as a solid "Plank" is one that is both challenging and fun!

The "Roll" teaches your body to be able to move into and out of positions with the abdominal brace in place.

Photos on the right illustrate an Elite level roll which can be done with any other combination of the Planks and Side Planks.

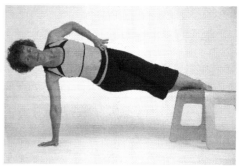
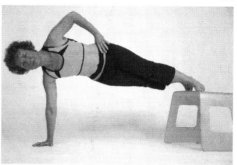
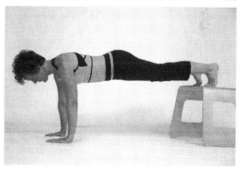
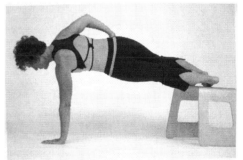
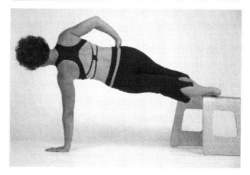

13. Conclusion

The possibilities of the human body are only limited by our inner restraints. The possibilities surrounding the Planks and Side Planks are similarly unlimited. I encourage you to be creative, to progress gradually and, above all, have fun.

Good luck with your core strengthening!

Acknowledgements

Iwould like to thank my clients who have inspired me to be creative in my goal to assist them in achieving their goals. Many of my clients have said to me that they always wished they could take their Physical Therapist to the gym. This book is an attempt to do just that.

I appreciate the support of my husband, Richard, who works countless hours as my photographer, camera man, editor, and publisher. I am blessed. His patience and dedication to our projects are the only reason they materialize.

For Kaitlin Cacciotti who stimulated the idea for this book. I supervised Kaitlin when she was a Kinesiology student. Thank you Kaitlin for listening to the initial ideas and your encouragement.

I am grateful to the many researchers and clinicians (the list goes beyond the reference list at the back of the book) who spend countless hours studying and advancing core training. You provide the foundation that allows professionals, such as myself, the freedom to explore what works in the real world knowing there is research data behind it.

References

There has been a lot of excellent research in the area of core exercise and its affect on fitness, back pain, and other conditions. I am fortunate to have been able to access and draw upon this material while developing this book. The following are the key books, lecture, and other publications that I have used.

Akuthata, Venu, and Scott F. Nadler. "Core Strengthening." Archives of Physical Medicine and Rehabilitation Suppl. 1 85 (2004): 86-92. Web.

Hodges, Paul, PhD. "Lumbo-pelvic Motor Control: Advanced Clinical Assessment and Treatment of Motor Control Dysfunction in Low Back Pelvic Pain." McMaster University, Hamilton. 2009. Lecture.

McGill, Stuart, PhD. Ultimate Back Fitness and Performance. Third ed. Waterloo: Backfitpro, 2006. Print.

McGill, Stuart, PhD. Low Back Disorders. Windsor: Human Kinetics, 2002. Print.

Santana, Juan Carlos, PhD. The Essence of Stability Ball Training Companion Guide. Boca Raton, Florida: Optimum Performance Systems, 2000. Print.

About the Author

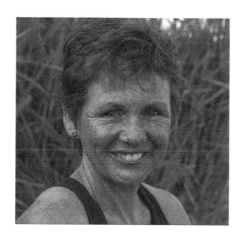

Margaret Martin is a Physical Therapist with over 28 years of experience helping individuals achieve their health and fitness goals.

She graduated from McGill University—School of Physical Therapy in 1984.

She teaches Yoga, Tai Chi, and Nordic Walking and is also a Certified Strength and Conditioning Specialist. Margaret has worked in a variety of clinical and industrial settings in Canada and the US.

Margaret combined her clinical Physical Therapy experience and her knowledge of fitness training to develop the *Building a Stronger Core* course for health and fitness professionals.

Margaret is the recipient of the **2011 Award of Distinction from the College of Physiotherapists of Ontario** for her achievements and significant contributions to Physical Therapy. She is the author of two books on exercise and bone health, *Exercise for Better Bones* and *Yoga for Better Bones*, and the creator of an online course for health professionals on osteoporosis treatment and management, *Building Better Bones*.

She is the proud mother of Katherine and John whose strengths go far beyond the core!

Her Physiotherapy and Personal Training studio, **Function to Fitness**, is located in Ottawa, Ontario.

Find out more about Margaret at: www.margaretmartinpt.com.